AF615748

HEALTH
and the
ENVIRONMENT

ONE LUNG TO GO

To Muller

5/26/03

Leonard Pay

HEALTH and the ENVIRONMENT

One Lung To Go

Leonard Pax

Rutledge Books, Inc.

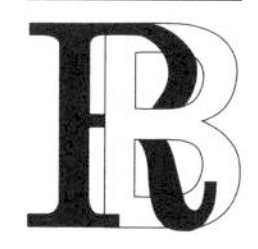

Danbury, CT

Rutledge Books, Inc.
107 Mill Plain Road, Danbury, CT 06811
www.rutledgebooks.com
1-800-278-8533

Manufactured in the United States of America

Library of Congress Cataloging in Publication Data
Pax, Leonard
Health and Environment: One Lung To Go

ISBN: 1-58244-085-9

1. Fiction.

Library of Congress Card Number: 00-103906

CONTENTS

INTRODUCTION

This is the story of Joe Darrell who lost his most precious possession, his health, as a result of the extended close contact with a fellow worker. He was in love with a beautiful model and had qualified for the engineering training program with General Motors, but failed the physical examination. His chest X-ray revealed that he has pulmonary tuberculosis, moderately advanced. This story gives a vivid account of the drama, romance and life in a sanatorium in the early 1940's. It is a story of a disease, tragic love, the struggle to regain health, and the problems encountered after release.

The doctor in charge of the sanatorium was a leading chest surgeon and participated in the advancement of medical science. However due to the fact that medical education, medical practices and legislation were inadequate for proper identification, treatment and control of tuberculosis, youth and society suffered the consequences.

These were trying times for the Darrell family. Joe's mother was committed to the sanatorium because of an improper diagnosis. She was pregnant. After three months she finally obtained an overnight leave and a physical from her doctor. In his opinion she never had TB, and in keeping with her promise she returned to the sanatorium, then left without permission.

Joe's fiancee had to spend several months of rest at home. Her parents would not allow her to visit with anyone. Their engagement was broken. A year passed before they met for a night out.

Less than fifty percent of the fellows who shared the sun-porch with Darrell recovered. After a year and eight months, he was released following sincere medical counsel. When he visited the GM employment office, he was advised that the training program would be too rigorous. He then decided to go to Arizona.

Hitchhiking on Route 66 he got as ride with an attractive gal in a 1940 convertible who was headed to California.

Chapter I

THE DOCTOR'S REPORT

It was early one February morning in the year 1942 when Joe Darrell parked his car and walked toward the factory gate. A high chain-link fence encircled the plant facility. This was wartime—two months after the attack on Pearl Harbor, 7 December, 1941. The factories took every precaution against sabotage.

"Good morning," he said to the elderly security guard who met him at the gate. "My name is Darrell, Joe Darrell; you have my identification."

"Mornin'," answered the guard, peering at him across the top of his glasses.

Darrell smiled. This was the opportunity he had strived to achieve. The small flakes of snow that floated about danced before him as he watched the guard step inside the small-framed office and search through the papers lying atop his desk. Darrell was eager to begin his training in the engineering course offered by General Motors.

The guard eyed him thoughtfully and said, "You don't have

any identification, but here's an envelope for you."

As he opened the envelope, he sensed something was wrong. What could be wrong? He wondered. He read the single line: "Report to the Doctor's Office". A strange puzzled feeling encompassed him. Again, he read the single line. Then pensively, he stuffed the note into the envelope and thanking the guard, he walked toward the office. The spring in his step was gone. The morning atmosphere that had once seemed so cheerful to him had changed to a gloomy gray, speckled with flakes of snow that floated about as if to warn him.

Inside the doctor's office a nurse directed him into a small room and told him to be seated. He remained there in the middle of the room. He took two steps forward and circled back. His blue eyes were clear but puzzled. When the doctor entered, he calmly greeted Darrell, and with a sedate mien, he pulled a large brown envelope from the filing cabinet that stood in the corner. He studied Darrell with a penetrating stare through his thick glasses. He asked, "Have you ever worked around a lot of dust, emery dust?"

Darrell shook his head and there was an awkward silence before the doctor continued, "Have you lost any weight or had night sweats?"

"I have lost a little weight."

"Take off your coat and step on the scale," commanded the doctor, pointing to the far corner where the scale stood.

After he had adjusted the weights, the metal arm balanced at 151.

"With your frame you should weigh more than that."

"I've lost about fifteen pounds," Joe replied thoughtfully.

"How tall are you?"

"Six even."

"How old?"

"Twenty," Joe replied. "Not quite old enough to vote."

In the pause of silence that followed, the doctor pressed a button and a fluorescent light flashed inside a cabinet. Then he thrust Darrell's chest X-ray under the clips of the lighted screen. Soberly, the doctor announced, "I think you have tuberculosis."

Darrell stood there in a daze. Many ineffable thoughts rushed through his mind: Was Pat all right? What about our plans for June? Our date tonight? It can't be. What would Dad say...and Mother...and my brothers and sisters? Are they endangered?

"Do you know of a sanatorium?" asked the doctor, interrupting his thoughts.

He nodded his head with thoughts of a friend, Bill Read, whom in his senior year of high school more than two years ago had been committed to a sanatorium. Also a year ago John Read, his father, who had worked next to him in the cost department, had broken down and had to return to the sanatorium after five years.

"Yes," he replied. "A friend of mine is in the sanatorium. He has been there about two and a half years. How serious is the infection?"

The doctor pointed to the X-ray film. "It looks as if there is a cavity here the size of a silver dollar. And here there are several smaller ones. It appears to be moderately advanced. It is serious."

Darrell took the large brown envelope that the doctor offered. He walked listlessly away from the doctor's office. With each step his heart sank deeper and deeper. He recalled the cough that had developed a year or so ago which he thought was a heavy cold, for it had disappeared and then came back again with another cold. Now, once in awhile his throat seemed to be irritated. A dry cough had slowly developed which he had attributed to cigarettes. He hadn't begun to smoke until he had graduated from high school in June of 1939. During the spring semester in a chemistry laboratory exercise a resultant reaction produced chlorine. The test sample had been slow in reacting and when he leaned over the small crucible to see, a sudden blast of yellowish green, suffocating gas caught him full in the face. He gasped for breath. The heavy pungent gas seared his lungs. The pain was sharp and cutting. Choking and coughing he had been led to the open window where he was told to breathe deeply. It hadn't occurred to him that his lungs might have been seriously damaged and it didn't occur to him now. He thought of the physical examination that he had about a year ago, and now he realized that it was too superficial. Other tests could have been administered and an X-ray taken sooner that might have provided earlier detection and prevented, or at least lessened, the seriousness of the infection. He was conscious now of the X-ray that he was carrying. What is to happen? He wondered.

"Pat, Darling, all our plans for the future are destroyed!"

The little flakes of snow were throwing soft white blankets over the cars parked systematically row after row as if they were trying to get in. He brushed the blanket of snow off the windshield with his glove, threw the large brown envelope on the seat, and started his car, a '38 Chevy that was half paid for. He drove automatically without much thought as to where he was going. Yesterday, Mr. Cregor, the personnel manager, had told him that this course was equivalent to a college degree and that from these graduates, the future executives would be chosen. Then, before he realized, he slid to a stop in front of his apartment. Inside he took his shabby suitcase from the closet and among the clothes was the fragrance of Pat's perfume. Turning toward the bureau by the window, he saw her picture and as he stared at her, she suddenly became real, laughing, talking, dining, and dancing; all the places they had been, the things they had done all came back to him. There were long wonderful evenings when they stretched out on the rug in front of her fireplace. In the darkened room, tongues of flames licked the air while howling wintry winds swirled snow against the dark windowpanes. Their faces glowed in the darkness. Lovely, beautiful lips mixed with sparkling champagne added to her gaiety and passion.

Pat Romane was Joe's age. She was a model in one of the more exclusive, uptown department stores. He had met her at a party last summer, and since then he had seen her quite often. All his plans had been wrapped up in her. He tried to think of a way to break the word to her, but the words wouldn't come. He looked at his watch; it was nine o'clock. He had to go to Patterson Field, which was adjacent to Wright Field and located about ten miles east of Dayton, where until yesterday he had been employed in the administrative training program as a stock tracer in engine repair.

At Patterson Field, Darrell received a temporary pass from the guard at the gate to go to the finance department to pick up his payroll check.

"Forty-two dollars and twenty-three cents," he said to himself. "My last check! That won't last long! Forty-two dollars and twenty-three cents!"

Slowly he walked toward his car, purposely avoiding engine repair. He didn't care to meet or talk to anyone now. About a month ago, while he was working, he had coughed up some blood-streaked phlegm and when he told the nurse, a big, buxom gal, she said in a sweet sarcastic tone, "Oh honey, go back to work. You probably have a head cold and it's coming from there. If you were hemorrhaging, you wouldn't be standing there. Here's a couple aspirin!"

It had only happened that day and he thought the blood probably did come from his nose. Anyway, he didn't feel any pain; so little did he know about the symptoms. They were hardly noticeable and too easily attributed to other conditions and ignored.

A B-24 crashed-landed and burst into flames on the field. With a shrill whining blast of sirens, two fire trucks raced across the field. Momentarily, he stopped to watch. The fire meant little to him; he had a tragedy of his own. As he drove away, he took a last look at Patterson Field where he had worked for the past eight months. He passed a squad of men on drill. What wouldn't he give to be one of them!

Returning to his apartment, he dialed RA-9764. A rapid "buzz-buzz-buzz" sounded in his ear and he let the receiver fall on the hook. While he waited, he placed the suitcase on the bed, opened it, and straightening the punctured side, gathered the loose clothing that was in the bureau drawers and threw them carelessly in. He shoved the bottles from the top of the bureau around the corners and among the clothes, leaving Pat's picture until last. He wanted to kiss her once more and run his fingers through her long black hair, but he couldn't, or wouldn't now! Again he dialed RA-9764.

"Hello?" purred a soft sweet voice.

"Hello," he responded, trying to sound cheerful.

"Hi, how are you?" replied Pat, all excited. She could always sound as if she was thrilled to pieces.

"Just fine," lied Joe. "Did you sleep well?"

He had left her house late last night, or rather early this morning.

"I was sound asleep when Miss Keeling called about ten minutes ago. Darn it. I've got to be at work by twelve-thirty today. A special showing or something." There was a note of haughtiness in her voice when she talked about the special showing for this was supposed to be her day off. "I feel so wonderful!" Pat continued. "How's the engineer?" She was turning on that subtle charm of hers that he liked so well.

"I'll tell you all about it in a few minutes."

"Oh great! Will you take me to work?"

"Yes, Darlin'."

"I've got something special planned for us tonight!"

Now we have special plans...that's just fine. "That's what I want to tell you."

"What is it?" asked Pat, interrupting, "Don't keep me in suspense."

"Something very important. I'll be over in a half-hour, or sooner."

"I'll be ready, but hurry, Dear! I love you."

"I'll hurry."

"But be careful. It's snowing."

Darrell returned the kiss that he heard as he waited for Pat to hang up. Slowly the receiver slipped through his fingers and came to a rest. For a moment he stood by the phone, dazed and suddenly exhausted. Pat would be deeply hurt. It had all vanished. The opportunity for a fine education, freedom and health, his most precious possessions, were all gone. Darrell tried to collect his senses as thoughts of his friend, Bill Read, who had spent more than two years in the sanatorium, ran through his mind. He wrote a note telling the landlady that he had to leave for the West Coast on an emergency transfer. No use telling her, he thought as he disconnected his radio and gathered the toilet articles from the bathroom. She always wanted to know too much about everyone's business and then broadcast it all over the neighborhood. At that time he didn't realize the seriousness or importance of informing those with whom he had come in contact. The apartment required a thorough disinfection in addition to a thorough cleaning. All too frequently neither was accomplished and the germs, including the tubercle bacilli that floated about, could cause many new infections.

Before closing the suitcase he placed Pat's picture on top of the clothes. The clothes on hangers he took as they were. He drove away from the apartment toward Pat's house as he had done so many times in the past. Pat lived about four miles away in the northwest section of town. It had stopped snowing. The avenue was slippery and dirty with the tread of tires, and occasionally the rear of his car slipped from side to side. Momentarily he forgot his troubles, but his subconscious mind kept repeating and repeating: "How to tell her? How to tell her?" Turning left off Salem Avenue onto the street where Pat lived, he saw the attractive homes with the neat lawns now covered with snow and people sweeping the sidewalks. It was almost eleven o'clock when he stopped in front of Pat's home and started up the winding walk that had already been swept. Pat rushed to meet him as he approached the terrace which had been shaded in the summer by a colorful blue awning where they first had kissed and now, under the gray sky in her mauve woolen suit, she was more attractive than ever. He took the black coat that she was carrying and held it for her. Then he straightened the collar and her long black hair, and waving to her mother who stood in the doorway, they started away hand in hand.

"Why so serious?" she asked, after waiting for him to speak.

Composed and quietly, he replied, "I'll explain on the way." Pat looked startled. This wasn't like Joe at all. She wondered what was troubling him. His carefree happy smile and even his consideration for her seemed to have disappeared. His blue eyes were cold and motionless as he held the door for her. She hesitated when she saw his clothes on the rear seat.

"Are you moving?" she exclaimed.

"Um...yes," he replied, closing the door.

When he rounded the car, she opened the door. "You're not like yourself. What has happened?"

"Pat, I've got some very disheartening news."

"It can't be that awful!" she said with all her charm, as if to add encouragement.

"It is," he said, pulling away from the curb. "I'll not be able to see you for some time!"

"What are you saying?" she gasped. "All our plans!"

The words echoed in heartbroken syllables.

"You don't mean that. What ever has happened?"

They were driving on Salem Avenue now, nearing the heart of town, as Darrell pulled over to the curb. There he told her of his talk with the doctor. His eyes welled up with tears.

"Pat, I couldn't take it if anything happened to you. I want you to have an X-ray taken, just to be on the safe side." As he was talking, his eyes fell upon the engagement ring that he had given her. "It has been wonderful. We have so many memories."

Tears formed on her dark eyelashes and rolled down her cheeks. He drew her to him. "Not that, Darling," he whispered as he brushed his fingers over her hair and held her until he could no longer think clearly. Finally he said, "It's time for lunch or you'll be late for work."

"I don't want anything to eat and I don't want to go to work."

"You'll feel better," he said handing her his handkerchief from the lapel pocket of his suit, "and no more of this."

The traffic moved along at a crawling pace. It had begun to snow again, more heavily than before. They stopped for lunch and by the time they left the restaurant, they had agreed to postpone their plans and their June wedding. They hardly spoke. Only an occasional comment was exchanged before they reached the entrance of the store where she worked. There the farewell was brief—a close embrace, no kisses.

The windshield wipers moved back and forth, swish...swish, as if repeating, all over...all over.

Chapter II

THE RETURN HOME

In his profound contemplation, he drove fast, much too fast on a snow-covered highway. The road was a familiar one leading home. Several times the rear of the car began to slide and he cut the front wheels into the direction of the slide. He misjudged a sharp curve and his speed. The car spun around and came to a stop on the shoulder of the road. He gazed down into the ditch alongside the highway and then at the large brown envelope that now lay on the seat beside him. The envelope and the sudden trip seemed like a nightmare. Fortunately there wasn't another car in sight as he turned his car around and continued homeward.

When he stepped out of his car in the barnyard, Buster, his dog, rushed toward him, barking and jumping, his whole body wagged with his tail from side to side. Buster leaped up to greet him almost knocking him down. Joe staggered back several steps before he regained his balance. Playfully, he grabbed his dog's huge paws and swung him around. For a moment his mind was free from the trouble that the future held. His mother was standing in the open doorway of the large brick house. A look of surprise and then, as always, a happy welcome smile greeted him. Joe gained courage, reached for the large brown envelope and proceeded up the stone walk that was covered with a thin layer of snow. It had stopped snowing and the air was cold and crisp. Mrs. Darrell drew the coat that she had draped over her shoulders more snugly about her neck—shoulders that were slightly inclined with the years of loving care given to her fourteen children. Joe was the second eldest. She stepped back as he entered. With her eyes fixed upon the envelope, she closed the door behind him.

"Do you have more papers to fill out?"

"Mother, I've failed to pass my physical exam." Then he paused and said quietly, "The doctor said that I'll have to go to a sanatorium!" As he spoke, a blank expression covered his mother's face. She turned slowly without any sign of emotion and silently led the way into the large dining room. When she turned to meet him, there were tears in her eyes, and as was her habit, she covered her left eye with her fingers.

He held up the X-ray for his mother to see. She stepped closer, peering at the film through checkmated tears.

"I can't tell very much about it, though it looks as if there is something wrong there—these white cloudy spots," she said in a hurt voice, pointing to them. Then she added in a whisper almost as if to herself: "TB!" Suddenly he remembered a cousin who had died from TB about fifteen years ago. There was a stigma attached to it. People didn't know how to cope with it. It was known as consumption and the plague, and it was feared. Public education and the precautions necessary to prevent the spread of infection were sorely lacking. Slowly, she sat down on the edge of one of the dining room chairs and staring at the floor, covered her left eye with her fingers again. When Joe was a little boy, he and his brother, Charles, had quarreled over a metal-edged ruler.

Mrs. Darrell had attempted to take the ruler away, but momentarily, Joe had held the ruler firmly. When he let go, the ruler flew up and struck his mother's eye. The sharp metal corner of the ruler had cut deeply into the eyeball and the left eye had been removed. She wore a glass eye, which was the same shade of green as the other, and uncomplainingly she continued to work, day after day, seven days a week, washing, ironing, mending, cleaning, and cooking. Her work was never finished.

Joe slipped the X-ray into the envelope. "I'll go to the sanatorium at Lima tomorrow and have it checked."

"Is Bill Read still there?"

"Yes, he is."

"And John Read, who you used to work with?"

"As far as I know, he is. I worked with him a year and a half."

"They've been there a long time and Bill's father was there five years ago," she said, slowly and pensively as she arose. Her straight brown hair was combed back and rolled tightly in a round knot. He followed his mother into the large kitchen where three little winsome tots were playing in one corner.

"Joe is home! Joe is home!" began the three little tots in chorus.

Occasionally he would bring candy home for them, but this time he had forgotten. He had been deeply absorbed with thoughts of the sanatorium. He had visited Bill Reed several times more than a year ago. It was so isolated and confining.

"You go ahead and play. Joe doesn't feel well," said Mrs. Darrell, quietly. Then she added, "I can't hear myself think."
The three little sisters stopped yelling. With happy dirty faces, mouths open, they stared at Joe, who was still wearing his overcoat.

Mrs. Darrell draped her coat across the rocking chair, paced across the faded, worn linoleum to the range, lifted one of the lids and said, "The fire is about out. No wonder I feel cold." Then she picked up the battered coal bucket that was filled with corncobs and poured some into the stove. The stovepipe extended above the metal warming closets and disappeared into a round hole in the chimney where the ivory painted wall had become brown and black with the stain of smoke. The oven door was open. When Joe was a little boy, he would climb upon the door to warm his back on the chilly wintry mornings. His mother was in her middle forties, sturdy, and in spite of all, she enjoyed life. She enjoyed working with Mr. Darrell and the family in the fields at harvest time, shocking wheat, shucking corn and picking tomatoes. Mr. Darrell called her a "rough and tumble gal."

"Joe, have you told Pat?" she asked.

"Yes," he nodded thoughtfully, and added, "I asked her to have an X-ray taken."

"What did she say?"

The kitchen door opened. Mr. Darrell, who had been out repairing the farm machinery in the barn, entered and said, "Well, I see the prodigal son is home." After the ironic remark, a big welcome smile wrinkled his cheeks that were red from the wintry air.

Joe smiled half-heartedly.

"You look as if someone stole your girl," said Mr. Darrell as he removed his leather cap.

While Joe was at home, Mr. Darrell had never approved of his working in town. Even while Joe was in high school, he hadn't approved of his playing basketball or playing in the high school band, because that interfered with the farm work. Mrs. Darrell had interceded and in the end, Mr. Darrell usually had given in to her. The muscles of his 160-pound, five-foot-eleven frame were hard from the long hours of work on the farm. The responsibility of feeding and clothing the family during the days of the depression had its effect upon him at times. Mr. Darrell had wanted Joe to do as he had done—stay at home and work on the farm until he was twenty-one.

It was Mrs. Darrell who broke the bad news. Her voice rang out strong and firm like a bolt of lightning through the dark stormy sky, only to falter and tremor on the word "sanatorium." Mr. Darrell removed his steamed-up glasses. His red cheeks became white. Joe shivered. Cold, blue and very solemn eyes pierced him from head to foot. So this is what happened while he was away from home. Joe had to work in town at the furniture factory. There he had worked next to John Read, who came down with TB a year and a half ago. Then he had to leave for the big city. Even while he was at home, often he had stayed out late at night. How is it that coughs sometimes lead into this consumptive disease and sometimes do not? Germs are present sometimes and sometimes not. The environment of the workplace was so important. Mr. Darrell shook his head. His voice was low, very low and somber. "Joe...Joe...Why?" And turning to Mrs. Darrell he asked, "What are we going to do?"

"We'll manage someway," she answered softly.

Mr. Darrell took out his can of dry crumbly tobacco—tobacco that he had raised on the farm—filled his corncob pipe and stood there by the table between two curtain-less windows. Joe related his heart-rending tale of woe. His future life was now a burden and a real disappointment to his parents. But parents were always hopeful as long as there was life. He had a strong physique, a good attitude and a will to do whatever was necessary to confront this silent enemy that had robbed him of his health. As he stared through the windows that overlooked an orchard bordered by a row of huge cedars where snowflakes nestled in the pine branches, he suddenly felt very tired. His mother filled the teakettle with water from the old-fashioned pump that stood over the sink next to the ceiling-high cupboard.

"The school kids will soon be home," she said, "and they'll be hungry and cold. I'll have to prepare some soup. Joe would you like some?"

"No," he replied, "I think I'll lie down for a while. I feel sleepy."

"Your old bed is still in the corner of Charles' room right above the kitchen," she said and added, "It's warmer there."

Joe left, went to the car, and took his suitcase and clothes up to his brother's room. A gloomy problem hovered over the house that was usually cheerful and noisy with the laughter and cries of children.

Chapter III

A SANATORIUM VISITED

The following morning he left for the district sanatorium at Lime, Ohio, about forty miles from home. The sun was high and the thin layer of snow had melted, only along the north side of the ditches lay patches that were hidden from the sun. There was nothing on his mind except the seriousness of the facts contained in the film of his X-ray. Driven by a compelling force, he entered the hospital grounds over a lonesome winding road bordered by brambly hedges and the well-kept lawns that were now a drab shade of green. The lonesome road curved and wound into a graveled parking area shaded by huge elms, which were now barren. To his right, a wooded bridge crossed at a narrow neck leading to a row of cottages. It made a beautiful setting, if such it could be for people like Joe Darrell, trapped in the tense drama of this old ivy-walled sanatorium.

The nurse he met in the hall entrance directed him to the clinic upstairs. He wandered up the cement stairs where a strange medicinal odor hung in the air. He moved through a dark, narrow, musty hall that creaked as he walked and past a closed door where five pajama-clad patients sat awaiting treatment. The door opened. There was a far away, long lost look in their eyes. A woman patient entered the clinic. The strange medicinal odor was everywhere. Further down the corridor an office door was open; someone was dictating letters. There behind the desk sat a doctor, clad in white hospital attire, opposite his secretary, a little elderly woman with a pad and pencil beside a typewriter.

The doctor continued dictating. His voice was strong and he pronounced the long medical words with full rounded syllables; words that Darrell had never heard before. Occasionally he leaned back in the swiveled chair and glanced up at the X-rays on the three lighted screens, or at Joe who stood there holding the large envelope at his side.

"Sign the letter, Doctor Sheridan, Superintendent," he said as he arose.

"What can I do for you?"

"Doctor," he said, raising the envelope, "I would like to get a report on this X-ray."

"Let's have a look at it," he said as he took the envelope.

After he had removed the three films, which he handed to his secretary, he thrust the X-ray under the clips of the lighted screen. A change of expression crossed the doctor's face and as he stared through his glasses at the film, his eyes seemed to grow.

"Is this your X-ray?" he asked, still staring at the film and taking several steps backward.

Joe nodded, stepping around to see.

"You have pulmonary tuberculosis, moderately advanced," said the doctor, stepping forward. Then pointing to the upper portion, he continued, "This is the upper right lobe. Here is a cavity the size of a silver dollar." He circled the white spot before he continued. "And here, one, two, three smaller ones. There is infiltration here in the left lung."

His eyes had followed the doctor's pointed finger upon the

film. He had spoken fast and Joe stood there in an enigmatical state as if he couldn't believe what he had heard.

Doctor Sheridan stepped into the corridor. "Miss Stevens, will you take a sputum check?"

Then turning toward Darrell, he asked, "Where was this film taken?"

"General Motors, Dayton, Ohio."

"More employers should require X-rays," commented the doctor who participated in, and followed, the advances made by medical science. It wasn't until 1940, after years of uncertainty, that mass X-ray screening came to be generally accepted by labor unions as well as management and the public. Union leaders were overcoming workers' objections to medical examinations. More labor contracts contained health clauses and a few began to specify chest X-ray as a condition of employment. It was a means of detecting early infection for the fortunate ones and provided some protection from dangerous exposure to others in particular the youth of the country who were more susceptible. Diagnostic tests were unable to detect the minimal signs of latent TB. There was no generalized test, such as a blood test, that could screen out those infected by the disease. Most doctors focused their interests in curing individuals, but did not deal in group or preventive medicine as such. A large proportion of the physicians were none too familiar with the latest diagnostic methods. Some of the private patients received less careful examinations, and attempts to control or eradicate TB were seriously handicapped by the inadequacies of medical education.

Miss Stevens, the laboratory technician, tall, slender and attractive, finally made her appearance carrying a small bottle. Doctor Sheridan nodded his head toward Joe.

"Can you raise anything from your lungs?" queried Miss Stevens in a southern drawl as she handed him the small bottle.

He coughed and cleared his throat of some yellow phlegm. The nurse took the bottle and left for the laboratory.

Doctor Sheridan, tall and heavy built, was now sitting on the edge of the desk. He was young, in his early thirties. He had specialized in the diagnosis and treatment of respiratory diseases. His entire life was devoted to the patients of this old ivy-walled sanatorium.

"I saw on the envelope that your name is Joe Darrell. Where is your home?"

"Celina."

"Do you know Bill Read?"

"I graduated in '39; a year before Bill."

"And did you know John Read?"

"I worked with him about a year and a half in the cost department at the furniture factory. I left there about a year ago."

"Very interesting...and how do you think you contracted tuberculosis?"

He shook his head as if he didn't know. There were so many variables and contributing factors of which he was not aware. Most important was the close exposure over a period of many months combined with late hours, improper diet, rest and exercise. His parents had warned him of the dangers, but he didn't heed their warning.

"Doctor," called Miss Stevens, leaning through the open doorway, "sputum positive."

The report sounded like a sentence. He wondered how long he would be in.

"Celina is in Mercer County, isn't it?"

Joe nodded.

The doctor contemplated. There was a shortage of beds and nurses. Sanatorium space was very limited and crowded. Much of it was taken up by advanced cases that should have been in the hospital. Finally he said, "We'll make arrangements to have a bed ready for you on Monday. You need immediate care. Mercer County has a bed open."

"How long will I be in?"

Doctor Sheridan thought of the consequences of what his reply might be. It was a concern of most new patients. He tried to instill into his patients as much hope for recovery as possible by creating mental peace and confidence. It was a chronic disease affected by all sorts of obscure factors.

"Eight to ten months," came the doctor's nonchalant reply.

Joe's voice echoed in disbelief and astonishment: "Eight to ten months!"

The doctor raised his brows and added a smile of encouragement, even though his thoughts were filled with an awareness of the long isolated months most of the patients had to spend. There were months of anguish when the patients were subject to all sorts of anxieties about their health and the future. And there were those who never recovered.

Joe turned away as the thought of eight months and his dreams of the future seemed to explode before him. He found himself walking along the barren ivy vines that clung to the walls as he listened to the low coughs that echoed therein. He didn't care to see or visit anyone.

It was late Saturday afternoon when he arrived home. His mother gave him a letter that had arrived with the morning mail. His eyes sparkled as he thought of Pat, but the letter was from Congressman Robert R. Pennington. Last year he had qualified for a first alternate appointment to the Naval Academy at Annapolis, but was not successful in getting the appointment.

He studied the letter. "It offers me another chance to take the qualifying examinations to the Naval Academy."

"Maybe you'll still have a chance later," said Mrs. Darrell, knowing full well that there could be no other opportunity.

That Saturday night he left home to forget the trouble he was in. He planned to see a movie, but in town he met a buddy of his, John Dibsby, a happy-go-lucky, handsome guy on leave from the Navy. Dibs, as Joe called him, had completed his boot training and was leaving Monday to be assigned sea duty. Dibs and Joe bought a fifth of bourbon before leaving Celina for the "Land of Dance", a nightclub in St. Henry. After nineteen miles they reached the crowded, smoked-filled club that was literally jumping with jive. Many of the men were in service uniforms and there were more women than men. The band was playing a tune entitled, Once in a While, and Joe thought of the time he had danced to that tune with Pat.

"...Once in a while, will you try to give one little thought to me, though someone else may be, nearer your heart..."

"No one will ever be nearer to my heart, Pat," he was saying to himself.

Dibs ordered a double bourbon and soda at the horseshoe bar, and a double with a water chaser for Joe. After the bartender had served the bourbon, Dibs raised his glass saying, "Here's to that last fling, Joe."

"To your health. It'll be a long, long time," he said, raising his double shot, "before we'll get together again. Down the hatch."

Then Joe ordered a round. A fellow sitting across the semicircular bar from Joe and Dibs, backed off the stool, lost his balance and fell flat on his face. The bouncer helped him up and staggered him out the door for fresh air as the four-piece band began to play, Rum Boogie, Rum Boogie, Woogie.

"Come on Matey," Dibs said to Joe, "I see a couple of hot lookers who are on the loose; a blonde and a redhead. You take the redhead and I'll take what's left."

"You go Dibs. I just don't feel up to it and I don't want to ruin your evening of fun. I just can't get with it. I'm going home early. Will you be able to get another ride?"

"Sure, but don't leave until I get back."

On their drive to the club, Joe had told Dibs about his affliction. "Bill Reed has been in the sanatorium more than two years. TB, that's really serious," Dibs had said. "But I'll be out in eight months," Darrell had said. "And I might still be able to enter the armed services, maybe the Air Force Flight Academy." He had wanted to enter last year, but his parents wouldn't permit it.

Joe took a sip of bourbon from the double shot glass. Reflected there was Pat, smiling just as always. Then her smile faded and there were tears in her eyes. "I'll never forget you, Joe," she was saying.

Then his thoughts drifted to Doctor Sheridan's words: "Eight months! We'll have a bed ready for you on Monday!" He just couldn't forget.

The four-piece band was now playing a tune that Glen Miller made famous: "In the Mood." It was one of Pat's favorites. Dibs and the blonde, who was wearing a red dress, danced to the beat of the drum and the blaring trumpet that grew louder and louder in a frenzied tempo. Couples jitterbugged around and swung out wildly, crashing into each other. With each crash he drew her closer, soft and warm, more and more exciting. The music stopped with a crash of the drum and the clash of the cymbals.

"I have a ride," said Dibs when he returned. "Are you sure you won't join us? She said you played center, opposite her brother, Jim Thompson, in the basketball tournament when we beat St. Henry High. She said that she remembers that one lucky, fall-away jump shot of yours that beat them in the final seconds of the tournament."

He gazed in her direction. There was a tantalizing gleam in her golden green eyes. His eyes lingered awhile on her cupid lips. Her flaming red hair waved against the light green dress as his eyes followed the low cut of her dress to the white, soft, inviting valley between her breasts. My, how she has grown—how radiant and wholesome looking, and how tempting. I wouldn't want to cause any harm to her, he thought. "Tell her that I'm not feeling well or that I have a previous engagement tonight."

Then Joe offered a toast: "Here's to it, and here's from it, and here's back to it again. If you're to it and can't do it, you may never get back to it to do it again."

Dibs raised his glass, then said, "To your health, Matey."

"When you get another leave, I'll be in better spirits and health," Joe said as he stepped off the barstool.

"Drive carefully," Dibs called to Joe as he left the nightclub.

Chapter IV

ADMITTANCE TO THE SANATORIUM

Darrell would never forget that Monday. He felt no pain, but he hadn't realized the seriousness of the effects of that restless Saturday night. Late Sunday he had coughed and hemorrhaged slightly. Monday he was in a sullen mood as he drove to the sanatorium through a slow drizzling rain. He accepted his affliction in a resolute manner and realized there was no alternative. Very few words were spoken by his dad, his mother, or himself. He parked the car under the huge elms near the ivy-walled sanatorium. Reluctantly, he cut the ignition and handed the keys to his dad.

"Take care of my car. I'll get out sometime, but I don't know when," he choked.

Then he took his suitcase from the trunk of the car, which contained the fifth of bourbon that remained after Saturday night. He also took a newly purchased pair of pajamas and robe, some toilet articles, and Pat's picture. Accompanied by his father and mother, who carried his radio, he started toward the steps, hatless in the chilling drizzle. His raglan-sleeved overcoat was snug and warm. From the top step leading into the hospital, he gave one last backward glance toward the car and the lonesome, open road that appeared so very inviting now. Take a good look Joe. It will be a long time, he thought, as the choking sensation in his throat seemed to increase. There were many places to go and many things to do. It simply couldn't end here.

Listlessly, they walked through the dark, quiet corridor toward the small reception room on his right. A nurse, neat in her immaculate white uniform, sat at the desk. When she looked in his direction, he introduced himself.

"Please be seated," she said in a quiet, friendly voice.

Then followed the usual routine questions for admittance about his personal and family history. Joe needed his mother's help to list the names and ages of his brothers and sisters. Of the fourteen children, he was the second eldest at age twenty. Fifteen or twenty minutes and many questions later, the papers were completed and signed, and the nurse suggested they go to the room to which he had been assigned.

Reluctantly, he reached for his suitcase, the battered one with the punctured side, and took only two steps before the nurse stopped him and relieved him of his burden.

"I'll carry that," she said in a polite but firm tone. Turning to his dad and mother she added, "You may come along if you wish."

Pensively, Joe mused to himself. Surely I'm not that weak. As he looked from his dad to his mother, they only smiled encouragingly. The nurse led the way through a wide corridor into a much narrower one, barely wide enough to pass another person, almost like a tunnel. The walls were dirty and yellow with age, accompanied by a sickening odor. And as they proceeded single file, only the creaking of the well-worn wooden floor broke the forbidding institutional silence, as if it resented their untimely intrusion. Soon they approached a large elevator, entered, and rode to the second floor. They followed the corridor to the left past four small private rooms called cubbyholes with their doors ajar. In each room the raffled, bulging covers of the bed indicated that someone occupied it. It was very quiet and that strange medicinal odor was everywhere. On his right, four huge windows overlooked the parking area, his car, and the freedom of the open road. The corridor turned left and the nurse opened the glass-enclosed doors of a sunporch that had been converted into a ward of five beds adjoining the four small cubbyholes that they had passed. In the far corner was a vacant bed. The windows were open and the room was cold and damp. The four fellows who occupied the other beds appeared to be asleep; they were all very pale and deathly still. Silent questions ran through Joe's mind. Are they putting me in here with these four sick guys? Is this to be my cell? How long will my sentence be? Joe couldn't believe that he was that sick. It was so very quiet. He wanted to yell or do something, but he could say nothing.

The nurse placed his suitcase on the chair at the foot of the vacant bed and began to check the lockers in the adjacent corner for one that was empty. Even though she was careful and considerate, several of the metal doors banged. She finally ended the drought of words.

"This is your locker. Do you have pajamas?"

"Yes," he muttered.

And then, for a moment, Joe gazed in bewilderment at the high bed with the little bench beneath it, forgetting all about his dad and mother. The nurse took the radio, which his mother was holding, and placed it on the stand by the bed. His dad was very grave and somber looking while his mother tried her best to smile.

The superintendent of nurses, Mary Boswell, who had ushered them to the room, spoke a few tender, well-disposed words to them as she moved about straightening the pillows and turning back the covers. Turning to face Joe, she said, "I will show you to the bathroom. You may change into your pajamas there and then go to bed. This is rest hour."

Patiently, she waited as Joe took off his overcoat and hung it in the locker. From his suitcase he took his pajamas and robe. He was careful not to uncover the bottle of bourbon. The wool robe was a deep blue—everything was blue now. Phlegmatically, he fingered the white fringe of the belt as he followed close behind the nurse. As if hoping to assist Joe, his parents followed him to the bathroom door. With a smile the nurse left, and for a few minutes nothing was said. Words were helpless now and eyes of kindness and sympathy took over. To Joe, his dad's hair, which was once thick and black, seemed to be thinner and grayer. Joe had once been his daddy's little boy, and he was wishing now that he could go back again. He had dreaded the thought of what his father might have said, since he had left home against his father's wishes, but he had met the issue with understanding never a word against him.

"Guess this is it," Joe said hesitatingly. "Don't know when I'll get home."

"We'll come to see you Joe," said his mother, "and I'll bake, especially for you, some date cake that you like so well. And Joe," she added with motherly affection, "try not to smoke so much. You really should quit."

"Don't worry about the car. Charles will help keep up the payments," affirmed his dad.

Joe tried to smile as best he could in reply. The car was in good condition. It had offered him a chance to get out and around with the girls he took driving through the countryside. Those were the happy carefree days.

"Write and let us know if you need anything," said Mrs. Darrell as they backed away and turned to leave.

Through slowly moistening eyes, Joe watched them as they walked dejectedly down the creaking corridor and disappeared around the corner.

Methodically, he undressed and stepped into his new pajamas with the dark floral design. His wool robe was warm, long, and very blue. He wore his shoes unlaced and shuffled back toward the sunporch. As he passed each bed, a questioning pair of eyes met his, but he said nothing. Inertly, he emptied the pockets of his suit, letting the contents fall on the bed. Then he neatly hung his suit, shirt and tie on hangers in the locker. His meager supply of toilet articles was placed on the top shelf. He shoved the suitcase with the bottle of bourbon in the locker and closed the door. He gazed at the articles that lay on the bed. Slowly, he counted the money-six dollars and thirty-four cents-all the cash he had to his name. Well he wouldn't be going anywhere for awhile. Opening the drawer of the nightstand, he tossed in the money, pocketknife, comb, nailfile, matches, and four packs of cigarettes. There were no pictures on the nightstands. He wondered why. With his foot, he pulled the little bench from beneath the high hospital bed, threw his robe over the chair, and sat for a moment on the edge of the bed as the other patients stared at him in silence. They waited for him to speak, ready to tell him of their horrifying experiences. But this was rest hour. They were forbidden to speak. The air was chilly. He kicked off his shoes and slid back, kicked his feet beneath the upper sheet and the covers, then tacked them up around his neck. The clean sheets were crisp and cold, and the bed was hard. He curled up facing the brick wall, away from the stares. His troubled mind wandered and drifted away only to bounce with alarm as the old elevator that was just beyond the brick wall started with a crash and a bang.

"Wake up, wake up, Mr. Darrell," came the voice of whomever was shoving his shoulder. "I want to take your pulse."

He opened his eyes and saw the brick wall. His head rolled sleepily to the side and his eyes closed again. A cold temp stick was shoved under his tongue. It felt as large as a shovel and his eyes opened. Miss Sharen, in her white uniform, looked down at him with a little likable smile and young sparkling blue eyes. There was a slight pressure on his wrist. Her hand was soft and warm. He could feel his heart beat. Occasionally, she glanced from her watch down into the faint smile of his saddened, blue eyes.

The sallow-faced fellows in the room came to life. At least they stirred a little as they removed the thermometers from their mouths, looked at them intently, and one by one placed them on their stands. All he could see on his temp stick were numbers and graduated markings. He had no cause to read a thermometer before. Randall, the fellow in the second bed from the door, coughed and reached for his sputum cup, clearing his throat.

Then after careful scrutiny, he closed the lid.

"They'll fix that, Randall," shouted Towers, a handsome blonde fellow who occupied the first bed in the corner by the windows, which faced the four beds lined along the wall.

"It's a-about time they do; they've been t-trying now for t-ten years," replied Randall with an occasional stammer in his dejected monotone.

"Aha, aha, aha-a," echoed Towers' galloping chuckle as he picked a cigarette out of the pack that laid on his stand.

Darrell watched in wonderment as Towers flipped his wrist sharply to put out the match, blowing a steady stream of smoke through his thin lips.

Miss Sharen entered, hurriedly collecting the temp sticks and recording the temperatures on the pad she was holding. When she approached the third bed she asked, "How is Mr. Skinner today?"

Paul Skinner moved his head slightly toward her. "Better today," he replied in a low voice.

Several nights ago he had hemorrhaged profusely. His mother had been called and she had remained by his side the following day and night. He was young, in his late teens, and his cheeks were hollowed and extremely pale. His dark brown eyes followed the nurse who paused momentarily as she read Darrell's thermometer.

"What's my temp?" asked Darrell.

"It's all right," replied Miss Sharen, though it was 100.2.

Questions, many questions entered Joe's mind. He wondered how much time each of these guys had spent in here. Ten years! Was Randall serious, or was he trying to be funny? He wasn't about to ask now as his mind kept twisting and turning in a nightmare of shaky nerves and half sleep.

Almost two hours later the clattering noise of a cart and the savory scent of food awakened him from his saddened mood and sleep-like trance. He looked at his watch. It was 5:10. A huge porter lumbered into the room and raised the head of Skinner's bed, then placed a small bed table over his lap. When the porter asked him, he nodded in approval and looking about, he saw that the other fellows sat up in bed, legs crossed before them. He soon finished the light supper and as he waited for the porter to remove the tray and lower his bed, he understood why everyone else sat up except for Skinner. It was fifteen minutes later when the porter returned.

He felt better, lit a cigarette, and began a conversation with the fellow in the next bed whose name he learned was Bunnigan.

"When I entered," Bunnigan was saying, "I quit smoking, but when I saw that the others smoked, it was hard on my nerves and I had to send to town for cigarettes."

There was a slight pause as the smoke bellowed forth. Bunnigan's light brown hair was thin and ruffled; his appearance and actions were sly and cunning. His eyes were shrewd and piercing; his long nose was slightly tilted and topped by a high forehead. He was about thirty years old and well built for a fellow taking a rest cure.

Bunnigan continued in his smooth even tone of voice. "I've been in about five months this time. Spent ten months in here a year ago and when my daughter was born, the doctor wouldn't give me permission to go home. I had a room on the first floor then, and as I was leaving by the rear door, Doctor Sheridan stood in the hall yelling, 'We're letting your lung out. You have adhesions. You might have a spontaneous collapse and die,' but I kept right on going, and he kept yelling, 'You'll die! You'll die!'"

After a pause he asked, "Will you have to take pneumos?"

"Pneumos?" said Darrell with a question. "I don't know."

Towers had slipped into his loafer shoes and had taken a seat in the metal lounge chair that stood by the windows opposite Bunnigan's bed. He was tall and slender, about six-two, and his blond hair was cut short like a crew cut.

"You know what they are, don't you?" asked Towers.

"Not exactly," replied Darrell.

"Well let me tell you," he continued with a chuckle. "Doc's got a needle about that long," and he held up a long, slender, index ringer. Then he added in a stern voice, "Doc's got you on a big stretcher, strapped so tightly you can't get away, then he jabs that long needle right through your ribs and pumps you full of air."

Bunnigan and Towers were roaring with laughter as Darrell looked dubiously about. Randall, who had shuffled toward the windows, leaned against the dresser with his elbows and remained there motionless, staring through the windows at the bare branches of trees in the distance and the gray sky, as if he longed for something lost. There were no bars on the windows, but without health there was no freedom. On the outside they were a burden and destructive to their families and friends with whom they had prolonged contact.

Of all the diseases, tuberculosis was man's oldest and most puzzling enemy. Until now there were no drugs found to be effective against its consumptive appetite. Tuberculosis, in its slow and silent way, was working all the time and had infected its way around the world. The disease struck hardest among young men and women in their prime, condemning many of them to an early death. Its victims included many famous people. Among them were: Robert Louis Stevenson, Charlotte and Emily Bronte, Frederick Chopin, Mozart, Voltaire, Balzac, Keats, Eugene O'Neill, and Henry David Thoreau. History offers many examples of celebrated families who were afflicted with it. Louis XIII and the French Royal Bourbon family died of galloping TB. His autopsy revealed extensive pulmonary cavities and intestinal lesions. Keats was heavily exposed to TB and the unfortunate circumstances of life. His brother Tom, the youngest, died in December of 1818 at the age of 19. Keats wrote in the spring of 1819: Youth grows pale, and spectre thin, and dies. John Keats died of TB in 1821 at the age of 26. Keats and Shelly symbolized the romantic and consumptive youths of the 19th century. For Darrell, this was just the beginning of a long struggle to regain, or partly regain, the health that had been so carefully but thoughtlessly lost. There was little else except bed rest, nutritious diet and hope.

When the laughter subsided, Towers asked, "How long did Doc say you'd be in?"

"Eight months."

They roared again. Towers, who was twenty-four years of age, asserted, "Eight months? I came in here a year and a half ago for a check-up! Aha, ah-a, I'm still here. About three years ago I was released from Mount Vernon, a sanatorium in the north central part of the state, after spending a year and a half to be cured."

"An apparent cure," said Bunnigan.

"Apparent hell! I never had a cure," exclaimed Towers with a note of irony, and turning toward Randall, who was now sitting up in bed as if he was trying to catch his breath, he queried jokingly, "How long have you been taking a cure, Randall?"

Randall was twenty-eight. He had spent three years here previously and then three years in Arizona where he had a relapse. A church in Arizona had given him financial assistance for awhile, but eventually he had to return home where his parents were able to obtain assistance from the county. "Oh, f-fo-four years this time," came his jerky tones with a shrug of the shoulders as if four years meant nothing.

At that instant, one of the glass curtained doors leading from one of the cubbyholes opened onto the porch and out swayed a skeleton of a figure. His bathrobe, girded securely about the waist, hung loosely on his shoulder bones. The seat of his bathrobe was worn thin from sitting. There were two large thread-bare spots in the rear. He swayed toward the end of the sunporch and took a seat in a metal lounge chair next to Towers. It was a wonder how he kept going and held together.

"When did you get in with this ill-fated fortune?" he asked, then gave a short hacking cough. His head jerked and his dry uncombed hair covered his eyes. He took a folded paper cup from the pocket of his robe, opened it, and with a plunking splash, hit bottom. After a critical examination, he chuckled,
"That's a good one," while his Adam's apple bobbed up and down in his long slender throat.

Before Darrell could reply, Towers spoke, "Transfusion, tell Darrell how you could spit red."

Through his small, sunken, toothless grin, Transfusion, as the fellows called him, gave a hideous laugh, then began, "I could run the hundred yard dash in ten seconds flat, and after the race one of my buddies would say, 'Go ahead Trans, show 'em how tough you are. Spit red for 'em.' Ha-a-a...I went to a doctor and he gave me pills for a stomach ulcer...Ha-a-a."

The comment of the big tough nurse at Patterson Field came back to him now when he had reported that he had coughed and seen blood. In a sweet tone of voice, she had said, "Oh honey, go back to work. If you were hemorrhaging, you wouldn't be standing there. It's probably coming from your head. Here's a couple of aspirin!" And what had been taught in health education courses? Certainly nothing substantial as to subjective evidence of TB or the characteristic physical disturbances that were really meaningful. He was working the night shift and sleep was irregular.

"Of all the doctors," continued Transfusion, putting his shoes up on the edge of the chair and drawing his knees up to his chin, "I happened to go to one of the quacks that didn't recognize tuberculosis. That was a good many years ago, about eight. I rode the rails across country—California didn't want me."

He paused while he licked his chops, then inquired, "You guys going to play poker?"

"Yeah, it's getting late," commented Towers. "We only have a couple years left and we have so much to do."

"When we get out," Darrell injected with a smile.

"Do you play?" asked Bunnigan.

"Thanks, some other time," replied Darrell who wanted some time to collect his thoughts after a trying first day in the sanatorium. It was almost unbelievable.

Towers arose. He walked erect, which made him appear taller then he was, and pausing by the foot of the third bed, he asked, "How do you feel, Paul?"

"Better," Skinner replied, brushing his hand through his dark curly hair.

"You'll soon be playing poker again," said Towers, turning to leave.

The three left the room as if they were climbing up a mountain; Towers in the lead, a head above Bunnigan who was stout and of medium height, a machinist by trade. Then came Transfusion who was an inch shorter, looking gaunt, spent and breathless. The shadows of night were closing in upon the old ivy-welled sanatorium. Skinner rolled his bushy head to one side. "It's a good thing you didn't ask many questions. These guys can really pour it on if you give them a chance."

"I re-re-remember an old, white-haired fellow by the name of Smith," began Randall from a sitting position on the edge of the second bed, one leg dangling over the side. "When Smith entered, he-he asked a lot of questions and visited most of the fe-fellows as he roamed the halls that evening." Randall paused to catch his breath before continuing. "Af-After the lights were out, he cried far into the night and when morning rolled around, he wasn't there. He packed up and left during the night. Never did hear what happened to him."

As he spoke, the sunporch took on a sinister appearance in the graying shadows.

"How did you find out that you had the bug?" asked Skinner in low quiet tones from the third bed.

As Darrell related his story, Randall turned on the lamp above his bed. The night nurse, Mrs. Kenny, who pushed a cart loaded with nourishment through the doorway, interrupted the conversation that followed. She greeted the new patient with a sincere and comforting voice as she distributed the half-pint bottles of milk.

"How are you, Paul?" she asked when she approached Skinner's bed.

"Better," he replied.

"You had a rough time," she commented, filling his pitcher with water.

The night he had hemorrhaged, Mrs. Kenny had watched over him like a mother until Mrs. Skinner arrived. She was a jolly nurse with a corpulent figure that bounced as she walked. Later when she returned to collect the empty bottles, she straightened the pillows and pounded them into shape, tucked an extra blanket at the foot of each bed, then opened the windows.

The cold night air moved in and the room became very quiet. Randall began to read his Bible. Darrell turned on his radio. Soft music came over the air and with each tune was a memory of the places he had been when he heard that melody, the friends he knew, the girls he danced with, and the things they did. Alone with Pat, embracing her tenderly, lovingly, searching for her lips, which parted under his touch, they lingered on the terrace until the last guest of that summer party had gone.

Bunnigan and Towers entered the room and turned on their bed lamps. Slowly, the fellows trudged to the bathroom and back again, with the exception of Skinner who remained in bed. Nine o'clock drew near and one by one the fellows pulled the cord that put out the light fastened to the wall above the bed. The dim light of the corridor gleamed through the half-glazed windowpanes; Darrell turned off his radio to forget his memories. He heard Bunnigan and Towers replay several hands of poker and heard muffled coughs that echoed through the stilled corridors, but in his heart there was sadness—a deep sadness born of the thoughts of all that he had lost. Pat was lost. He couldn't help but feel the tears, tears that wouldn't run away, but remained there until they were choking at his throat. No one ever experienced a deeper sadness as thoughts of this day and the days to come ran rapidly through his mind. They couldn't keep him here. He wouldn't stay here. At last sleep, a much-welcomed sleep, moved in on his thoughts and his thoughts vanished into nothingness.

Chapter V

THE FIRST DAY

The click of a lock startled Darrell. Mrs. Kenny, the night nurse, tip-toed softly into the room, closed the windows, and turned on the radiators. She then gave Skinner his wash water. Darrell looked about. A cold gray dawn was breaking. Towers, Randall and Bunnigan lay snuggled deep and still beneath their blankets. Skinner, with sleep in his eyes, was trying to brush his teeth. The radiators hissed and clanged. Darrell closed his eyes, and all was quiet again.

"Good morning, everybody," shouted a cheery voice, and a smile beamed from her face as Miss Sharen bounded about in a lively manner. She took their pulses, shoved the temp sticks under their tongues and left the room. Skinner curled up and went back to sleep. His temp stick hung loosely from the corner of his mouth. Randall began his slow shuffle to the bathroom.

Dishes clattered in the corridor. It was a few minutes after seven as they were served breakfast in bed. When Darrell was working, he seldom got up in time for breakfast, which was so important for proper nourishment. Now he didn't have to get up for breakfast.

Skinner grumbled as he shoved a bowl of oatmeal aside.

"Oats, feed it to the goats."

Darrell ate all his breakfast: the oatmeal, although he hadn't cared much for it before, a soft boiled egg, two slices of toast that were almost cold, tomato juice, milk, and coffee. Then he lit a cigarette and joined the straggling procession to the bathroom. When they returned, his eyes followed the network of suspended pipes. For now, white canvas curtains were drawn around Skinner's bed. Towers held his nose while commenting, "Bedpan Alley." Then he opened the windows wide.

"Towers," shouted Miss Sharen, "this is bath day." And while struggling with the shaky knobs to rewind the windows, she lectured, "Just because you're in class three and can take your own bath, do you want to freeze the fellows?"

Towers was at a lost for a fitting comeback at the moment. He laughed sheepishly, then said, "Bedpan Alley!"

"Darrell, did you ever get a bed bath?" asked Towers when the nurse had left the room.

"No, I'm looking forward to it. I can hardly wait."

"Your bed will look like a tent," he continued.

"Omar the tent maker!" added Bunnigan and they roared with laughter.

"What's going on in here?" questioned Miss Sharen, pushing a large gray hamper of soiled bedclothes into the room. "Get some music on your radio, Towers," she commanded, ignoring the laughter.

Towers dialed to a program called Do You Remember- a program of hit tunes of the past like the one that was playing now.

"...We are poor little black sheep who have lost our way, Bah, Bah, Bah..."

Yeah, Darrell thought, I sure lost my way...don't know why I had to end up here...What a place!

"...Lord have mercy on such as we. Bah, Bah, Bah...."

Miss Sharen had already begun to give Randall his bed bath when another nurse entered carrying a basin of water. As she passed, Towers gave a low whistle. There was a slight smile on her lips as she greeted Skinner, then set the basin of water on his stand.

"Miss Downley, that's Mr. Skinner, who can be nice when he wants to," said Miss Sharen, who was washing Randall's leg. Then she added, "That whistle you heard was Mr. Towers."
Miss Downley turned, soaping the washcloth as she glanced at Towers who nodded a greeting.

"This is Mr. Randall," said Miss Sharen, "and in the bed next to Skinner is Mr. Bunnigan, another one of the wolves, and in the corner, a new patient, Mr. Darrell. He still looks a little down-hearted, but better than yesterday."

There was something about her youthful figure that reminded him of Pat Romane—the firmly curved lines under her white nylon uniform; impulsively he winked. Only she noticed the sadness that disappeared momentarily.

As Miss Downley continued to wash Skinner's chest, Darrell noticed two round red scabs, and leaning toward Bunnigan, he whispered, "Say, what are those little round scabs on Skinner's chest?"

"Remember when Towers talked about that long needle?"

He nodded as Bunnigan paused.

"Well," he continued in a whisper, "that's the evidence. He gets pneumos on both sides."

"He does!" exclaimed Darrell as if he couldn't believe it.

"Yeah, he does," affirmed Bunnigan in a matter of fact fashion as Miss Sharen placed a basin of water on his stand and yanked on the covers.

Darrell had just taken off the top of his pajamas when Miss Downley approached saying, "Hold the sheet tight; I'm going to pull the covers off."

With a jerk the sheet slipped from his grasp. He made a hurried grab for it.

Her startled look changed to a smile. "I thought you had your pajamas off," she said. "I can't give you a bath that way."

Darrell removed the bottom of his pajamas under the cover of the sheet as the fellows roared.

After the nurse had finished washing and drying his arms, she drew the sheet and towel down across his hips.

"Is this your first day?" he asked as the washcloth moved in and around his navel.

"Oh no, I've been working in surgery more than a month." As she held the sheet, he rolled over on his stomach. She had a rosy clear complexion and there was a warm glow in her light brown eyes. He wondered why she had selected a place like this. She had taken her nurse's training at St. Rita's Hospital in Lima where she had met Doctor Harman who had worked in the emergency room, occasionally to help out, as did Miss Sharen, for there was a shortage of nurses and doctors. They were both in love with Doctor Harman.

"Will you be working on this ward now?" he asked.

"Occasionally to help out, and on the women's ward. Roll over," she commanded.

He twisted and rolled over on his back again. "I hope it will be more often than that."

"I do too," she said as she uncovered his leg and placed his foot in the basin of water. Her fingers tickled around his foot in search of the washcloth. His toes curled as the washcloth wiped its way across the sole of his foot and around his toes, and then, gradually around his thigh up to his hip. The touch tingled and there was a blush of excitement through his entire body.

She handed the washcloth to him saying, "Finish your bath."

The nurses made up the beds. There was an air of cleanliness when he climbed between the crisp unwrinkled sheets. It was morning rest hour from nine until eleven. They were permitted to read or listen to the radio, but not to talk. Darrell lay staring into an immense, gray wintry sky that stretched far beyond the electrical wires and the barren tops of the elm trees that encircled the sanatorium.

The afternoon rest hour, two hours of complete rest from one until three, was enforced. The fellows weren't permitted to talk, read, or listen to their radios. Darrell slept, and when rest hour was over, Miss Stevens, the laboratory technician, shoved a wheelchair into the doorway and entered carrying a small black bag. She was tall and slender, and wore a ready smile for everyone. Unknown to most of the patients, she had taken treatments and spent a considerable amount of time in a South Carolina sanatorium.

"Mr. Darrell, the doctor will see you in his office," she announced in a soft southern drawl. "First I'll need to take a sample of blood."

She took his blood pressure, then jabbed a needle into his forearm, hit the vein on the first try and drew out a small test tube of blood. Then she pierced the tip of his middle finger and a couple drops of blood fell upon the glass slide. As directed, he climbed out of bed and walked toward the wheelchair past the row of beds; he stared questionably at Randall whose slender fingers turned to the page that had been marked with a red ribbon.

The narrow red ribbon made the tan paleness of his hands more pronounced and his dark brown eyes peered intently through the brown rimmed glasses set high on the bridge of his pug nose. He continued to read his Bible without looking up. Randall's breathing was short and heavy. Ten years spent taking a cure! Darrell thought as he seated himself in the wheelchair. It was strange to be wheeled away. No exercise was permitted now.

Leaving for the office, Miss Stevens stopped and said, "You all save your sputum cups tomorrow mornin' for a check."

In the room across the hall from Doctor Sheridan's office, Miss Stevens clamped his identification numbers on the black X-ray screen. After his X-ray was taken, an intern, Doctor Harman, set his black bag on the long adjustable stretcher-like table. Hurriedly and silently, he glanced through the papers that had been filled out when Darrell had entered. Then, as he spoke a few words to Darrell, he pulled a chair and a stool alongside the table.

As he was directed, Darrell seated himself on the stool that faced a large window overlooking the parking area. The probing stethoscope was pressed against his back, up and down, left to right, around and around. He wondered what the doctor could hear. Then dull hollow thuds of the doctor's rapping finger echoed in his ears. Doctor Harman handed him several folded tissues saying, "Cover your mouth with these, then exhale and cough."

The probing stethoscope pressed against his back again and the doctor said, "Again, until I tell you to stop."

He thought it would never end. Then as directed, he whirled around on the swiveled stool and the process began on his chest all over again. A healthy chest retained the same sound or precussion when the breath was held after a deep inspiration. The use of the stethoscope had become the symbol of medical practice; it was helpful in examining the chest for auditory behavior. Following his chest examination, he was carefully examined from the tip of his head to the bottom of his feet. He had never received a check-up like this before. It was now too late for preventive measures.

At length, Doctor Harman said, "We'll begin your pneumothorax treatment tomorrow. Air will be induced into your pleural cavity to rest your right lung. The infiltration in your left lung should clear with bed rest. You need complete bed rest."

"How long will I have to have complete bed rest?"

"There are twelve classifications," began the doctor, "ranging from class one through class twelve. Class one denotes complete bed rest. We'll assign you class one and a half, which permits you to go to the bathroom once a day-outside of that, complete rest. After you have had several negative sputum checks and cultures, you'll be raised to class two and then you'll be permitted to go to the bathroom as often as necessary. In class three you may take your own bath. In class four you will be permitted to be up one half hour, and so on through the classes to regain strength and to test and prove that the tuberculosis infection has been arrested." There was a slight pause. "You will most likely need complete bed rest for a year or more." Again there was another pause. Doctor Harman was a young and handsome intern who had completed his medical schooling in Canada and had attended some specialized courses at Ann Arbor, Michigan, where he had met Doctor Sheridan and Doctor Putner, a renowned chest surgeon. He was slender, about five foot eleven inches, and very thorough in his work which he enjoyed. He also enjoyed the friendship and love of two beautiful nurses, Gloria Sharen and Mary Jane Downley. When his internship was finished, he would return to Canada to serve in the medical corps assigned to the Royal Canadian Air Force. The doctor continued, "Do you have a girlfriend or girlfriends?"

"Yes," he said. "I was engaged to be married in June."

"If you haven't, you should write and tell her to have an X-ray. Also advise your friends and close associates, and the people you worked with, to have an X-ray taken."

"What about the family?" he asked and wished now that John Read had informed him.

"Your family will be advised."

That evening he wrote a letter to Pat, telling her about the general routine of the sanatorium; the fellows who shared the sunporch with him; the nurses, Gloria Sharen, June Stevens and Mary Jane Downley who reminded him of her; and, as best he could, about the coming pneumothorax treatment. He asked about her X-ray and informed her that the doctor said he had to have complete rest for eight months to a year, but he told her that he hoped to be released in eight months and hoped she could visit him soon. He wanted to telephone, but there were none available to the patients and they were not permitted to use the office telephone. It was all so strange and sad, this life in the sanatorium. All these things he expressed in his letter to her on this first day in the sanatorium, the first complete day. The windows were open wide, nine o'clock drew near, and one by one the bed lamps became dark. In the silent night, the night nurse adjusted the windows as the cold air of the night moved in while youth and beauty were on the wing.

Chapter VI

PNEUMOTHORAX TREATMENT

A big fellow, with shoulders stooped to a huge bay window, sauntered onto the porch carrying a little brown kit. Gray hair fringed the back and sides of his bald head. Darrell seemed to be the first he noticed; they exchanged glances—a surprised glance, then behind it a disappointed stare.

Beanball, as the fellows called him, hooked his razor strap to the round pin of one of the door hinges and stood there strapping his razor in a lackadaisical manner as he stared about.

"Does he expect to get a shave?" he asked. The fellows laughed. They knew Beanball, who talked tough, acted tough, and looked tough as he leaned over them holding a straight edge razor.

He brushed the lather into Randall's beard with a few circular motions of the left hand. Then with long sweeps of the razor, the fastest shaving that he had ever seen, the heavy stubbles snapped and cracked as they were whisked away by the scrapper. Then Beanball left and returned in a few seconds with Randall's washcloth, supposedly hot.

"Nothing but peachfuzz," he said as he passed Skinner's bed.

Bunnigan's beard wasn't as heavy as Randall's and his shave was even faster.

Then with a swish of his hand across Darrell's beard he said, "I don't know whether I ought to shave you or not."

Once while he was shaving Darrell's face, there was a sharp nick under his chin, which began to bleed freely. He paused momentarily. "Oh-o-o, I nicked you a little."

It was more than a little. Beanball left and soon returned with a wet washcloth. He moistened a small white styptic pencil and applied it to the cut. The biting sting checked the blood. As soon as he had finished, he strolled through the door with his little brown bag. Darrell rubbed his chin. It felt as if his skin had been peeled away by the scrapper. The fellows laughed. It was morning rest hour. He waited nervously, yet patiently, for his pneumothorax.

At ten o'clock a porter wheeled a stretcher alongside of his bed and told him to take off the top of his pullover pajamas. The clothing hung to his chin and twisted at his elbow. Laughingly, Miss Downley, who had followed the stretcher into the room, offered her help and the top slipped slowly away. Her touch was warm, but he shivered in the cold air as she guided his arms into a surgical gown. After he crawled onto the stretcher, the nurse covered him with a blanket and tucked it around his shoulders. As the ceiling glided directly above him, Bunnigan called, "Don't stick too many holes in him."

The guffaw of the fellows rang in his ears and as the stretcher turned, the walls and the ceiling swung around and dropped down as he rolled under and through the doorway into the forlorn corridor. He was wheeled faster now, past the four large windows on his left and the four cubbyholes on his right. After a few more turns, through a much narrower and darker corridor, the stretcher, the ceiling, and the walls came to a halt. The medicinal odor was everywhere, but he hardly noticed it anymore. A few pajama-clad patients, seated awaiting treatments, talked in low voices. He heard the voice of John Read and his head rolled to the side facing him. A shocked hurt expression covered John's face.

"Joe Darrell!" sounded the startled voice of John Read. "You here? What happened? How long have you been here?"

"Hello, John." The days that he had worked next to John Read were very real in his mind. How could he explain what had happened? He noticed that his hair was now white as snow. "I never thought that this could happen to me or that I'd be here.

Can't hardly believe it. How's Bill?"

"Doing better now. He should be released this summer."

"I'm getting my first pneumo today. Are you waiting for a pneumo?"

"No, I'm supposed to get an X-ray this morning. I can't take pneumos anymore because my lung stuck to my pleural wall. I took pneumos for five years and then they gave me a phrenic.

There was a puzzled, questioning look on Darrell's face.

"That was six months ago," Read continued. "The phrenic nerve which controls or innervates the motions of the diaphragm is crushed so as to be temporarily put out of commission affording necessary rest for the lung. It can only be performed on one lung, one side of the chest at a time, and will usually last from eight to twelve months before the diaphragm on that side becomes active again."

"How long have you had tuberculosis?"

"I was gassed during World War I and several years later my trouble started."

God, that was a long time ago! What a terrible thing to happen, he thought. It never occurred to him that the gas from the high school laboratory test could have effected his lungs. "How are you doing now?"

"I'm in class twelve. I ought to be out in couple months if everything goes well."

A tall middle-aged nurse with glasses on the low hump of her nose interrupted and wheeled Joe into the clinic. There she leaned over him as she drew the blanket down to his hips, telling him to roll over on his left side. Doctor Sheridan finished washing his hands at the small sink and dried them with the sterile towel that the nurse had handed him. He then moved up behind Darrell and selected a spot between the fourth and fifth rib with his middle finger that exerted pressure in a circular movement tickling his ribs. The small hypodermic needle sent warning waves of hurt nerves waving at his brain, telling him to move away. Unconsciously, he raised his head to the sharp piercing sting.

"Keep your head down," demanded Doctor Sheridan.

He could go nowhere. The stretcher was solid and hard. The Novacain chilled and numbed the selected spot, then a much longer needle—not as long as the one Towers had described—pierced the welt left by the smaller needle, and bored down swiftly under the sensitive fingers of the surgeon. It moved slowly toward the protective pleural wall.

"Don't cough now," warned the doctor, and with a sharp sting the needle pierced the pleural wall.

The adapter of the small rubber hose joined that of the needle and air was forced into the pleural cavity. The bright red liquid in one of the vertical gauges bobbed up and down as pressure began to build within his chest.

"I bought a pony yesterday for Janie," said the doctor as he held the needle between Joe's ribs.

"Oh, I'll bet your little girls like the pony," said the nurse, staring out the window that overlooked a grove of barren maple trees.

Nervous perspiration that had formed under Joe 's armpits now trickled down across his chest. The bright red liquid climbed steadily in the gauge and as the pressure continued to increase, he wondered whether or not the doctor and the nurse had their minds on what they were doing.

"Janie is seven. She isn't afraid to ride," continued the doctor, "but Betty, who is five, screamed when I held her on Nancy, that's the pony's name...Ha, ha, ha-a..."

Joe thought that he would never stop laughing. The pressure increased in his chest and he wanted to yell out, "Get your mind on your work."

At last the doctor declared, "450 cc's. That'll be enough."

Joe heaved a sigh of relief as the needle was pulled out and released the vise-like grip of his right hand on his left as the doctor painted his pierced side with methiolate. He patched it with collodion and added a little dab of cotton that he rubbed around and around, leaving it there to seal Joe's punctured side. Then the blanket was drawn up across his shoulders and two swinging doors swung open as he was wheeled into the doctor's office that adjoined the clinic. The mounted pressure on his right lung was like a brick wall. Low voices whispered through the open doorway from the corridor where other patients stared in at him, said nothing, and when their names were called, passed by like flat tires after air. He was glad it was over, but tired of lying on his left side. Twenty minutes later, Doctor Sheridan entered.

"How are you, Mr. Darrell?" he asked, peering down at him.

"I feel an awful lot of pressure around my lung."

The doctor took Joe's pulse and replied with a smile, "You're all right."

When he arrived at the sunporch, Towers laughed and peered down at him. "They brought him back alive."

The porter grabbed him around the shoulders and Miss Downley lifted his legs. His shoulders were off the stretcher when suddenly the porter lost his grip. Darrell made a quick grab for the bed while the nurse hurriedly helped him to hang on as the porter wrestled him up. She straightened his surgical gown and covered him. He had almost lost his pajamas. Her touch was warm and friendly. In a sweet but firm tone of voice, she warned,

"You aren't permitted to sit up."

He gave the nurse a sweet smile in return, although he had almost fallen to the floor.

"Remember the fellow whose shoulder puffed up this big?" asked Towers holding his cupped-shaped hand three inches above his shoulder.

"He was in misery," added Bunnigan as he sealed the letter that he had written to his wife.

Miss Downley shook her head; her light brown hair brushed across the white collar of her uniform. "You guys," remarked Miss Downley, leaving the room.

Darrell waited and waited. Now is the time; the coast is clear, he thought. Carefully, he reached for his urinal that stood on the shelf of his stand hidden under a faded gray cloth. Under the covers with his knees raised, he placed the urinal.

"Miss Downley, Darrell wants to see you!" called Bunnigan.

The nurse hurried toward his bed. "What is it?" she asked.

The thought of the urinal embarrassed him. "I didn't call. Bunnigan is only fooling," he managed to say.

Bunnigan, Towers and Skinner roared to high heaven. Even Randall began to laugh, and under the covers he held the urinal for fear it would spill.

When the nurse disappeared into the drug room, he slipped the urinal from under the covers.

"Nurse! Nurse!" yelled Towers.

Alarmed and befuddled, he looked toward the door and in his haste, the urinal caught in the covers, tilted and partly spilled on the edge of the bed. The fellows bellowed louder than before and he saw Miss Downley approaching, trying to hold a sober face.

"Look what you've done!"

"It slipped," he said. He could feel the blood rush to his face, but he was thankful that it didn't spill on him.

The nurse took the urinal that he was still holding and placed it on the shelf of the stand. "You're supposed to remain quiet," she warned.

"Yeah Darrell, you should hold it," said Bunnigan.

"I'll be back to change your bed clothes," she said, ignoring the comment.

"It had to happen while she was on duty?" bantered Bunnigan after the nurse had left.

"That'll give him a chance to have his bed changed while he's in it," remarked Towers who desired more of her attention.

Slowly, Darrell was becoming more acquainted with the daily routine of the hospital and his new friends. When they were asleep, they appeared as innocent as angels, but when they were awake, the jokes were mostly on him since he was the newest member of the group. He accepted their wisecracks and found them to relieve some of the tension. He enjoyed their company and he joined in the discussions—discussions about the books they read, industry, war, religion, and TB. It was everywhere around them. It was in them, this ill-fated fortune that was his. He was beginning to realize that it would be some time before he would be released. He ate all the food that was placed before him, whether he liked it or not, and to relax, he tried to forget the things that were once such a vital part of him. All opportunity for active participation in athletic sports was gone. Plans for the future had to wait. He was conscious now of the importance of health. That strange medicinal odor seemed natural now. The sight of Doctor Sheridan, who nearly always made his daily rounds visiting the patients, was an added comfort.

"Good Morning! Good Morning! Good Morning!" said the doctor as he approached the end of the porch.

It was the fourth day for Darrell—the day following his pneumothorax.

"How do you feel today?"

"I feel a lot of pressure and pulling in my chest," replied Darrell.

"A-ha, probably have some adhesions. We'll fluoroscope you and give you another pneumo tomorrow."

Rubbing his chin he turned and approached the foot of Randall's bed. "I can't understand why you're still positive."

Randall was glum and sullen.

"I'll give you a phrenic on your left lung, that ought to help you."

"Th-That won't make me short of breath will it, Doctor?" queried Randall, who was receiving pneumos on both lungs.

The doctor looked solemnly at Randall. "A little perhaps, but it shouldn't bother you. You have some large adhesions on that upper lobe of your right lung and it appears as if your positive sputum is coming from there."

The description of adhesions made Darrell shutter. He dreaded the consequences.

Randall stared questionably. He was already short of breath. The doctors had tried, but were unable to cut his adhesions.

"I won't crush your phrenic nerve as much as I usually do, then your phrenic won't last as long."

Towers waved his classification card as the doctor turned. "It's four weeks today, Doc."

Doctor Sheridan's expression changed. A brief smile crossed his face as he marked the card with a four, raising Towers one class, permitting him one half-hour up each day in addition to his bathroom privileges.

"We'll move you to the new building one of these days."

A large grin widened his straight narrow nose. "I've waited more than a year and seven months to hear that."

"How was my sputum check?" asked Bunnigan.

"Negative," replied the doctor in a quiet voice, and added, "We'll see how your culture turns out."

Before Darrell could speak, the doctor raised his finger saying, "Positive. Stay in that bed." Then he pointed his finger at Skinner and emphatically said in firm tones, "You were positive. Stay in bed."

Skinner's face reddened. He grinned and nodded his head as if to say, I've heard that many times before. Skinner was beginning to feel more like himself again.

When the doctor left the room, he stopped at the nurses' desk and examined several charts. One was Darrell's. He was satisfied with what he saw. Darrell's temperature was down to normal and his pulse was regular. However, Darrell wasn't comfortable as the pressure in his chest seemed to increase. Pneumothorax was the best method, which was available at that time for resting a diseased lung, and had been accepted by American surgeons around 1912 based on good results reported from Europe. Since there were no effective drugs available, it was used except where the lung adhered to the pleural wall as had happened in John Read's situation. After five years he had a relapse. With some other diseases a person will develop some immunity and be relatively safe for the rest of his life, but a person who has had active tuberculosis is far more likely to have it again than one who has never had it.

Chapter VII

SUNDAY VISITORS

The footsteps that echoed through the corridors announced the approach of Sunday visitors. The fellows combed their hair and straightened their stands. For Darrell, it was his first Sunday in the sanatorium after six perplexing days. In the interim, he had received his first and second pneumos, and awaited his third.

Unknown to him he had large adhesions on the upper right lobe and was slated to have his adhesions cut. His infection was more serious than at first anticipated. He had written a letter home and another letter to Pat. He had seen Miss Downley only once—and that was for not more than five minutes—since the day that she had changed his bed. Miss Sharen, who was the regular nurse in charge of the surgery ward, performed her work with cheerful care.

The afternoon rest hour was over and Darrell watched an elderly couple parading slowly into the room. Mrs. Skinner was three steps in front of her husband who wobbled along behind and took a seat in the metal lounge chair that stood by the dresser. He nodded to his son, Paul, and Mrs. Skinner gave him a box of chocolates.

Skinner's eyes gleamed as he opened the box, eyed the candy, and then began to munch the velvety chocolates.

Mrs. Skinner stared at Darrell. Finally Paul, with his mouth full of candy, introduced his mother and father.

"Um-m this is...er...Joe Darrell. He's from um-m...Celina."

"Paul, you shouldn't talk with your mouth full. Celina? We're from Coldwater. That's seven miles from Celina," said Mrs. Skinner as she offered Joe some candy.

"Take another piece," said Mrs. Skinner. "There's plenty to go around."

Then she passed the candy around. Bunnigan declined because he was a diabetic. Randall took several pieces and Paul Skinner's eyes nearly popped when Towers took four upon the insistence of Mrs. Skinner, who flitted about bedecked in a blue coat with a big furry collar. The fur was the shade of her gray hair, fluffed in small curls around her head. When she returned the half-emptied box to Paul, he eyed it with a silly grin.

Bunnigan's wife entered. Quietly she said, "Hello." She then passed Mr. Skinner who was rocking back and forth, back and forth. His huge bushy head of curly gray hair bobbed as he unzipped his old leather jacket that was tight fitting. Then he patted his belly that hung over his belt. He was contented and remained silent as Mrs. Skinner, who stood by her son's bed, did all the talking.

A tall, red-faced man, about six-three or four, who must have weighed 240 or more, entered. The sleeves of his Sunday suit wrinkled at the elbows and the creases of his trousers sagged at the knees.

"How are you, Gene?" he said in a low sober voice as he wound his large bony fingers around the iron bedpost by Randall's feet.

"M-Much the same," came the dull monotone as if Gene was tired of answering the same question. "Did Mother come along?"

"She's still visiting the girls, but will be over soon," said Mr. Randall, staring down at his son who braced himself with his hands, then scooted back against the pillows and crossed his legs.

"How are they?"

After a moment of contemplation, his dad replied, "Mary Alice is doing well. She was negative on her first, or rather her recent, sputum check. Ellen is about the same and I guess you've heard about Bertha."

Gene shook his head silently.

Good God! thought Darrell. Four from one family in here! And he wondered, Why so many from one family? How could it happen? With medical care available, preventive measures and precaution, was Gene responsible? Casual association, he was told, is not serious or to be feared, as in smallpox, but constant exposure is dangerous, as had happened to him when he worked next to John Read. He thought of his brothers and sisters. Were they endangered? He had been away from home more than a year and his visits home were short and infrequent.

"Bertha received her initial pneumo Friday," continued Mr. Randall in solemn tones. "She had a spontaneous collapse. I talked to Doctor Sheridan. He's doing all he can."

Joe braced himself against his elbows and raised his head off the pillows as his mother and father approached. He wanted to get up to greet them. A strange helpless feeling possessed him.

"We received your letter," said Mrs. Darrell with a smile, handing him a green wrapped package.

With a curious grin, he unwrapped the package.

"They're size C," she added as he held the pajamas before him.

"Norma picked the pajamas," said Mr. Darrell as he unbuttoned his heavy black overcoat.

"She said you would like the blue and gold ones, your high school colors. Norma is a cheerleader for the high school basketball team," remarked Mrs. Darrell proudly.

He held up the wide, red and gray stripped ones.

"Norma said they would help to cheer you," added his mother.

What a bright red! he thought, nodding his head in approval. Then he leaned back against the pillows as his mother glanced curiously about as if she had never seen the room. She leaned over him and whispered, "Isn't it crowded in here?"

The sanatorium was indeed overcrowded, like all others. There were over 400 TB hospitals and sanatoriums in the United States; however, in 1940 came the Draft Act and more and more beds were required to care for the rejected inductees who were found as a result of the mass X-ray screening. There was a sense of emergency, which made more urgent the search for therapeutic agents.

Mrs. Randall had joined her husband and Gene told her that he was still positive, and that on Wednesday, Doctor Sheridan would give him a phrenic. "I-I'm afraid the phrenic will shorten my breath some more," he continued. '"M-maybe I can take it."

"The doctors ought to know," said Mr. Randall.

Mrs. Randall grabbed her husband's arm. "I hope so. If only there was something more that could be done. We feel so helpless," she said.

In 1940, research had began for soil antibiotics that might be effective on diseases like TB which were beyond the reach of drugs already developed, such as penicillin and the sulfa drugs. And so there was hope. It had been more than ten years for Gene. Mrs. Randall had hope, but worried wrinkles lined her forehead. Her brown rimmed glasses were like Gene's and her nose was slightly pudged like his. Her straight brown hair, lightened by streaks of gray, was tucked up under an old-fashioned, felt hat that had once been in style in the late twenties, and her coat was a worn shade of brown.

Everyone had company except Towers who was visiting one of the women patients down the corridor from the sunporch on the surgery ward. Mrs. Skinner was still talking and Mr. Skinner was still rocking back and forth. Mrs. Bunnigan was seated beside her husband. Her long dark hair hung loosely around her shoulders and her hazel eyes gleamed as she talked about their little girl.

"She can say Mommie and I'm teaching her to say Daddy, but she can only say, Da-da. She looks more like you everyday. Her eyes are a sandy color now and her hair is lighter too."

Mrs. Darrell took a letter from the worn leather handbag that Mr. Darrell had given her on their tenth wedding anniversary in the pre-depression days. "Here's another letter from Congressman Pennington about your Naval Academy appointment," she said, handing the opened envelope to him.

"Is that all?"

Mrs. Darrell nodded.

"Didn't you answer his first letter?" asked Mr. Darrell.

"I meant to, but what's the use now? I mean there's no chance for that appointment now. I might get out of here in a year, if I'm lucky."

Mr. Darrell waved his calloused hand in added emphasis. "You ought to thank him for his consideration."

"I'll send a letter to his office later today or tomorrow."

"The county health doctor was out to see us," said Mrs. Darrell, changing the subject. "We had to fill out more papers. Everyone will have to have an X-ray taken. Maybe we'll all end up here!" she added with a laugh.

Mr. Darrell glanced out into the wintry sky. Little flakes of snow fluttered by the windows. "We won't be able to drive very fast going home. We drove your car today. It runs good, better than ours."

"The long drive is good for the car, like exercise for the body. I've been here a week and already I feel as weak as a kitten by just lying here," he said. There was a longing for the exercise and the good times that he remembered so well. He was slow to realize that there could be no more for a long, long time.

"You'll soon feel better," said his mother, and added, "We'll have to go. The little ones are waiting in the car and they'll be cold."

"You know how it is on the farm, Joe," his dad continued, "the livestock has to be fed and cared for, and Charles wouldn't like it if he had to do all the chores, especially on a Sunday night."

Mrs. Skinner walked out with them, exchanging comments, while Mr. Skinner remained seated, rocking back and forth.

Mrs. Skinner returned from a tour of the ward and Mr. Skinner stopped rocking, leaned back in his chair, took out his large pocket watch and said, "It's about four-thirty, Ma. Time we go."

"Paul, you must eat better," said Mrs. Skinner, and to Bunnigan and his wife who were passing she remarked, "Aren't leaving are you?"

"I'll be around a few more days," replied Bunnigan.

When the visitors had gone, Bunnigan returned in a slow shuffling gait. "Paul Skinner, you and your father didn't say more than five words to each other all the while he was here." A sheepish grin covered Skinner's face. His protruding ears grew red and he stammered for words. "Well, we did enjoy seeing each other and being together."

Bunnigan laughed aloud. "All the two of you did was to stare at each other and nod your dumb heads."

Late that evening, Darrell wrote a night letter to Congressman Pennington, and when the nurse was passing out the evening nourishment, he gave it to her to send. It was her first night on duty. She read the telegram back to him with a southern drawl. The nurse, Eve Stevens wasn't at all pleasant like her sister, the laboratory technician. She held a straight, frozen face.

Bunnigan had stopped reading his book. "Ho, ho-o," he bellowed. "That's the best one I've heard. After you've been in here a week, you send a wire to let him know that you won't be out as soon as you thought. Ho, ho-o, as if it made any difference. Ho, ho-o-o."

Eve Stevens' lips parted with a half-smile as she stuffed the telegram into her pocket and walked away in a stately manner saying, "You all want any oil tonight?"

Darrell's eyes followed her from head to foot and foot to head.

"What a build. She's really stacked," commented Bunnigan after she had left.

Transfusion swayed onto the porch as he did almost every evening. He took a seat in the metal chair, drew his knees up to his chin, and began clapping his gums about a fellow on the first floor who had been bellowing his lungs out.

As the loud resonant coughs continued, Darrell asked a silly question, or so it seemed, "What's wrong with him?"

The fellows burst into laughter. Transfusion replied, "That's crazy Red Baylor coughing for a hypo and the nurses don't think he needs one. Doc hasn't prescribed any for him."

"This is no place for a cough!" added Darrell.

Amid the deep bellowing that continued, Bunnigan left the room to join Miss Stevens in the drug room. The coughing that re-echoed through the night grew fainter and fainter. Shortly after the lights were out, Bunnigan tip-toed to his bed.

"Well, did you make any progress?" asked Darrell.

Bunnigan ignored the question. "We were discussing some of the latest books. She is well read."

Two days later Joe received his third pneumo—550 cc's of air. While he was fluoroscoped that morning, Doctor Sheridan told him that he had large adhesions on the upper lobe of his right lung. This meant one thing—pneumonolysis—cutting those adhesions, if possible. His surgery was scheduled for the following week when Doctor Putner, a renowned surgeon from Ann Arbor, Michigan, would be available to perform the skillful operation. According to the fellows, there would be wide leather straps to hold him to the stretcher and sandbags would be piled around his chest. Then Towers said that the surgeon would drive a wedge between his ribs. Strange as it may seem, he waited anxiously for his scheduled surgery. "If that's what the doctor ordered, let's have it! The sooner the better," he said to himself. "Anything to get out of here." There wasn't any alternative at this time. It was one step on the road to recovery, a big serious one. Success was in the surgeon's capability.

The following day Randall received his phrenic. The orange disinfectant solution that had been painted on one side of his neck extended up to his ear from under the small bandage that covered the incision at the collar bone. Several times during the day, he was forced to sit up in bed to catch his breath and he read his Bible more fervently. Darrell was saddened as he watched his struggle for breath that continued endlessly.

Late that evening, Doctor Sheridan, on his way to pay Randall an unexpected visit, hesitated as he rounded the corner that approached the sunporch. His eyes focused on Eve Stevens and Bunnigan in the drug room. With an eye upon the open doorway and an arm around her waist, Bunnigan pointed to the shelves lined with pills. "Quick," he whispered, "give me a chew-up."

A puzzled look crossed the nurse's face.

"Don't look. There's Doc. Give me the pills," he demanded in a whisper.

The nurse reached for the bottle and gave him two chew-ups. "Is there anything else tonight?" she drawled, keeping her voice well in control.

Bunnigan crunched the chew-ups as he looked into the glaring eyes of Doctor Sheridan who towered over him in the doorway.

"Hello, Doctor," he choked, trying to swallow. Then his face flushed as he squeezed by the doctor.

"Miss Stevens, the patients aren't permitted in the drug room," announced the doctor.

"Yes, Doctor. It won't happen again."

"See that it doesn't," he added in a warning tone of voice.

"How do you feel, Randall?" he asked, approaching his bed.

"A-A little short of br-breath," he replied with a frown.

"You'll get over that in a couple of days. I'll have the nurse give you a couple of sleeping pills," he affirmed. He had Miss Sharen's report of Randall's shortness of breath and he hoped that he would soon improve. As another alternative, he would lessen the amount of air induced on Randall's next pneumo in order to give him more breathing capacity.

Randall had a restful night, but early in the morning Bunnigan hurried out of bed in a fast shuffle toward the bathroom. The windows were black in the pre-dawn hours and only an occasional cough and rattling snore disturbed the stillness.

The chew-ups were working.

The March winds roared in with the approach of Darrell's scheduled pneumonolysis. Frequently throughout the day, Randall sat up, braced himself with his arms, and gasped for breath. Darrell signed a paper that granted Doctor Putner permission to operate and on the eve of surgery day, his chest was shaved as the howling blasts of wind wailed through the barren tops of the elms and whipped around the barren ivy vines that clung to the brick walls.

Chapter VIII

DARRELL'S CHEST SURGERY

The morning atmosphere, tense and shackled, welled up within Darrell. He reached for his glass of water, but it wasn't there. He had received nothing to eat or drink since last night and there was an empty feeling in the pit of his stomach. His radio began to buzz, crackle, and pop.

"Why the static?" he asked.

"They're cutting adhesions," replied Bunnigan.

"Man alive! That was a big one!" jeered Towers.

"Do they use electricity to cut 'em?" queried Darrell.

Guffaw followed. "Sure they do. Listen to that static. There goes another big one."

Miss Sharen entered carrying a glass of water and a small paper cup that contained two yellow capsules and two small white pills. "Take them now," she commanded as she handed them to Darrell.

As she watched, he swallowed the pills and gulped the cool water.

"That'll be enough. Do you want to get sick?" asked the nurse, reaching for the glass that was now almost empty.

As the radio continued to buzz intermittently, he grew sleepy and began to drift into a relaxed mood as if he were on a cheap drunk. Through the corridor a stretcher rumbled. Someone else was returning from surgery. He thought they were after him and as the pendulum of time swung to and fro, he drifted dreamily, thinking of nothing in particular except the operation that flashed before him.

An orderly shoved a wheelchair into the doorway as Miss Sharen entered with a white surgical gown draped across her arm. Her voice flowed in smooth even tones. "Take off your watch and the top of your pajamas and slip into this."

He swayed on the edge of the bed, his legs dangling over the side. He looked at his watch as he laid it on the stand. It was about ten o'clock. Time meant little to him now.

"Do you have any false teeth or bridgework?"

"No," he replied with a smile that showed his even white teeth, but when he began to unbutton his pjs he needed her help. After the nurse guided his hands into the sleeves of the surgical gown and draped his long blue robe over his shoulders, she asked, "Can you walk to the chair?"

"I'd rather dance," he replied with a laugh.

Amused, the nurse steadied him as he swayed past the fellows who were enjoying the circus and joined in the laughter. In the surgery room, at the East End of the first floor, two nurses greeted him, their faces half masked. One was Miss Downley, and with a twinkle in her eyes, she assisted him to the stretcher under the glowing lamps and the white ceiling. He was surrounded by the whiteness of the blank walls and upon a lighted screen was his X-ray that had been taken yesterday.

"This will be cold," said Miss Downley, showing him a slab of shiny metal, which she then shoved under his left side.

He heard footsteps and voices in the corridor. It was Doctors Sheridan and Herman and others he could not recognize. The nurses were working faster now. Two small sandbags were piled against the front and back of his chest. Then a white sheet was draped over several rods making a screen before his face, and wide leather straps were drawn securely across his chest, waist, hips, thighs, and ankles. He tried to move, but could only wiggle his toes. Miss Downley peered in under the screen with a smile while Doctor Harman was strapping his arms back over his head. Then he took his pulse and remained there by his side. Doctor Putner, who was leaning over him, applied a pungent disinfectant that trickled in cold rivulets across his chest.

"Close your eyes," warned Miss Downley.

The pungent fumes stung his nose. Much pressure upon his chest followed a dull coldness, just as Towers had said, as if someone stood there driving a wedge between his ribs, the thorascope forced its way between the third interspace.

"Does it hurt?"

"I feel a lot of pressure."

"You're bound to feel pressure. We can't help that."

More pressure followed. It felt as if his chest was crushed.

"Look at the light color of this lung," said Doctor Putner.

Footsteps shuffled around to have a look-see. What could it mean? He wanted to see too. He opened his eyes and saw Miss Downley peering down at him and managed to smile faintly.

"Relax now. This won't take very long," said Doctor Putner in a commanding voice.

A wave of current shot through his chest with a ripping sensation. His muscles quivered, trying to let go.

"Relax, we're cutting inside your chest and we don't want to cut your lung."

Darrell pondered: Does he think that I want my lung sliced? How can I relax with that strong, shocking current?

"I'm trying to relax," he blurted, "but I have no control."

"Feel as if you're falling through the bed," said Doctor Sheridan.

I wish I could, he thought. A fat chance I'd have falling through this bed.

The surgeon waited, then tried again.

Again, he quivered and trembled with the current that shot through his chest.

The surgeon straightened. "These muscular guys have that trouble. Let's try that other cathode."

Again Doctor Putner tried, and this time the ripping sensation was like a tickle that snipped its way through the elastic fibers. "There was a short in that other cathode," he said when the snipping had stopped. "But, look at this one. I don't know if I can cut it."

Footsteps milled around to have another look-see and time began to drag. An ominous quiet prevailed. Miss Downley looked down upon him. He wasn't one open to prayers. Please, please, help him to cut it, he silently pleaded. Please, dear God, help him. It was so very still. Finally, there was a long, drawn out buzzing and snipping followed by the short ripping sensations and then the release of pressure. A cord in a suture pulled and tickled its way in stitches. The anesthetic was wearing away and he felt the last of the dull punctures made by the needle. A small bandage covered the incision and over this, wide bands of adhesive tape were securely strapped around to the middle, in front and back of his chest. There was a smile in Miss Downley's eyes as she removed the screen.

"Glad it's over?" she asked, removing her mask, the sandbags and the leather straps.

"Yes, it feels good to be able to move again," he replied as he kicked his legs to see if they were still there.

Doctor Putner stared down at him dubiously through blurry eyes. He said nothing. It had been a long morning. This had been a difficult one, touch and go. Soon the stretcher began to roll and he closed his eyes. Onto the sunporch, happy faces greeted him and he was carefully laid in bed. The dinner trays were already being served.

"I'll feed you in a minute," said Miss Sharen, cheerfully.

Although he felt tired, he didn't believe that he couldn't feed himself, but he was thankful for her cheerful help. With each spoonful the food grew larger and larger. He shook his head tiredly, sipped the milk and coffee through the bent glass tube that the nurse held for him, and soon fell into a restless sleep. When he awoke, he was hot and feverish.

The three o'clock pulses and temperatures were taken. He focused his eyes on the thin magnifying line of his temp stick. It read one hundred and one. He felt all the worse.

The nurse on duty, a big buxom blonde, commented, "Miss Downley said that you looked like a Mexican jumping bean."

Amid the laughter of the fellows, he replied, "There was a short in that cathode."

"You know, those doctors could electrocute a guy," taunted Bunnigan.

The nurse glared at him with her light dusty eyes snapping. "You know better than that."

She left, and after awhile reappeared with a bottle of rubbing alcohol. When she was giving Bunnigan his backrub, she practically emptied the bottle on his rump. "Oh, it slipped!" she exclaimed almost with glee.

Bunnigan let out a war whoop, holding his rear. It was funny, but Darrell couldn't laugh for fear he would hurt his side.

He could hardly laugh, but the thoughts of using a bedpan forced him out of bed. When he straightened, the tape pulled tightly across his chest and he shuffled along, one foot then the other. Nearing the bathroom door, Miss Barnes, the big buxom nurse, spotted him.

"What are you doing? Your chest is all raw inside! Your adhesions were cut."

"I don't want to use a bedpan."

"You'll hemorrhage! You'll hemorrhage," she protested wildly.

"I may as well go all the way. I've come this far."

"Well I declare," she said, placing her hands on her hips, feet wide spread and offering no assistance.

When he returned to the room, she was waiting with that wide pose of hers. "I'll have to report this to the doctor."

"It's done now and the walk felt good," he retorted.

He spent a restless night lying in one position, flat on his back, afraid to turn over. Once he awoke, alarmed by gnashing, grinding teeth. Good Gosh! Are there rats in here? he wondered as his heart began to pound. The rasping noise stopped and he heard Bunnigan smack his lips and mumble: "Blub...blub...I'll raise you...Sandbagging...Blub, blub...." Joe lay his head back on the pillow. Again there came the rasping "g-r-r-r" of teeth, and through the light that gleamed from the door, he could see Randall sitting up to catch his breath, his head nodding with sleep. That night a soft layer of snow had fallen and the air was clear and clean. Skinner stood by the window staring longingly at the blanket of whiteness.

"Good morning," echoed the voice of Doctor Sheridan from the corridor.

Skinner's protruding ears perked up and a second, "Good morning," echoed nearer. In a hurry, his long skinny legs bounded for the bed.

Amid the laughter, Doctor Sheridan stepped into the doorway. He took three steps, then stopped. His eyes grew large and his mouth dropped open. Skinner's face grew red, as red as his pajamas. The laughter stopped when the Doctor shouted, "Skinner, after all you've been through and all we did for you just one month ago, do you want to hemorrhage again?"

In the silent moments that followed, the doctor shook his head.

Darrell wondered whether Miss Barnes had told him about yesterday when he got up to go to the bathroom.

"Stay in that bed," he barked at Skinner.

Mary Boswell, the superintendent of nurses, stood behind the doctor and smiled amusedly.

He paused at the foot of Darrell's bed, shaking his head again. "You were a lucky boy."

He felt much better to hear that. It was consoling. He smiled in return. But after the doctor had left he pondered. Lucky, for what? To be here? To get my adhesions cut? To remain in this bed? How weary it becomes.

The following morning, Doctor Sheridan's fickle finger pointed directly at him when he barked, "Stay in that bed," His round cheeks puffed and his eyes glared like those of a bulldog as he continued, "or you get empyema."

Darrell was dumbfounded. The doctor had said nothing about bathroom privileges, which he continued to enjoy. Before he could gather his senses, the doctor was out of the room with long strides.

"Boy, you sure got it," said Bunnigan as if it were a big joke. "One day you're lucky and the next day you're getting empyema. Ho, ho-o."

"Empyema. What's that?"

The room became very quiet.

"Empyema is...a, a...when fluid develops in the pleural cavity and becomes infected with bugs," replied Bunnigan

"Is Doc telling me that because I got up yesterday?"

Calm compassionate eyes met his inquiry. It was no laughing matter and there were no answers.

"Do you think the doctors saw any indications when they were cutting my adhesions?"

"Perhaps," said Towers, and added, "Jim Carson has had empyema for years. He's the tall lanky guy down the hall. He had several stages of ribs, but that didn't stop the bugs, and since then he's had his side laid open five or six times and the pleural wall scraped or parts of it cut away. He comes in here for two or three weeks and then goes back to work. He always wears a bandage because his side drains."

He shuddered at the very thought, afraid to move. Later when Miss Downley visited him, her words were cheerful and kind, and he forgot the troubles that faced him, at least for awhile.

The following morning Darrell rode to the clinic in a wheelchair as did Randall and Skinner. Four women, seated in the folding chairs that lined the wall adjacent to the clinic, stared at him as he swayed passed them toward the end of the short corridor where three fellows sat opposite a wicker lounge occupied by two younger women. He hesitated as he approached them. For a moment he thought he recognized one of the girls. She glanced up at him, smiled, then she turned swiftly toward him. Her brown velvety eyes sparkled as she moved over to make room for him.

"Joe Darrell!"

"Hello, Betty," he said is a rather quiet surprised tone.

"I hardly knew you in that long blue robe."

"I hardly know myself," he said, seating himself beside her. His arm brushed against the smooth texture of her quilted robe.

"It's been a long time since I've seen you."

"More than a year," commented Betty Gordon, reminiscently, her head resting atop the back of the wicker lounge.

He turned toward her and studied her face that tilted toward him. Except for a brilliant shade of lipstick, she wore no make-up. Faded freckles dotted her cheeks and nose. She was thinner now.

"How are you?" he asked.

"Doc should raise me to class six soon," she answered, crossing her legs. The light green robe parted and draped from her knees showing the muscular form of her legs hidden beneath red polka-dot pajamas.

"How long have you been here?"

"Ten months," she replied as if it had been an eternity. Then her face brightened. "When summer comes, I'll be up in class and I'll be able to go walking."

He was wondering whether or not he would be up in class by then. They had met at a high school band concert at Coldwater where she played clarinet. He had played sousaphone in the Celina Immaculate Conception High School band, and occasionally the band director would ask him to help out at concerts and in the marching band at some of the football games. During some of the night games at half-time, the lights would be turned off and the band would march with battery lighted instruments. It all seemed such a wonderful experience and so long ago. "Me too," he said, turning toward her, "I'd go walking with you."

She thought of the night they had danced together at the "Land of Dance" after a football game years ago. She liked the soft tone of his voice, his profile, and his clear blue eyes that smiled in search of her reactions. Her face flushed and became vivacious. "Not very far from here," she said, "there is a large park bordered on one side by a golf course and a small lake. We could..."

Doctor Sheridan rushed around the corner followed by Doctor Harman.

Joe's eyes followed Betty Gordon as she marched through the narrow doorway. He had hoped to visit her as soon as he felt better and he wanted to get her room number.

When the women filed out, the fellows proceeded through the X-ray room toward the opposite entrance. Darrell waited momentarily. A fat women squeezed through and Doctor Harman said, "We'll have to put you on a diet." After a pause and a glance in Darrell's direction, he said: "Keep moving. Time's a wasting."

Darrell felt weak and hesitated as Betty Gordon approached, and there was only a faint smile as he brushed past her and entered a small room where Doctor Sheridan stood behind a sliding screen extended from a heavy metal cabinet. Nine fellows crowded in and around to the side and behind the doctors. When the doors closed, the room became pitch black and the screen flashed green with a buzzing sound. From behind the doctors, Joe peered curiously at the skeleton framework and the internal structure, but through the darkness he couldn't see who stood behind the screen.

"Turn around, Randall," said Doctor Sheridan, who could identify the patients by a glance at their lungs. The projected greenish rays of the fluoroscope faded away and Randall turned around in the darkness.

Darrell listened to the doctors who talked in low voices as the screen lit up again. "This is the troubled area," said Sheridan, pointing to the upper lobe of his right lung. "These adhesions are too large to be cut. Sniff, Randall," he commanded.

When Randall sniffed, his diaphragm on the left side moved up and down while his diaphragm on the right side, that had raised two inches since he had received the phrenic, remained stationary.

"You have a good phrenic, Randall," remarked Sheridan. "It should help you."

When the buzzing stopped, another fellow felt his way through the darkness past Randall, and as the screen lit up, a slender skeleton frame was visible. Two dark saclike masses hung partly collapsed.

"Due on the left side today, Skinner?" asked Sheridan.

"Yes," he grunted.

Feet shuffled around in the darkness. Darrell was the last to stumble along the metal cabinet. Pinned against the cabinet by the screen, the reflected rays cast a green shadow on the doctors' faces.

"Who is this?" asked Harman.

"This is Darrell," replied Sheridan. "Raise the screen a little."

The screen swung up and banged him on the chin. His head snapped and bounced off the metal cabinet.

The fellows laughed.

"Sorry," said Doctor Harman. "Turn your head sideways."

"Good pleural space," commented Sheridan. "Give him about 500 cc's today."

He grew weaker as he stood behind the fluoroscope. Six weeks in bed and his surgery had weakened him, Perspiration trickled from his armpits and grew cold along his ribs as the screen flashed on and off before him. Black and white spots whirled and danced, pressing down upon him like a hundred stars. The tape pulled and itched across his chest. The door opened and he dropped into the nearest chair where the fresh air revived him. Revived, he shuffled into the corridor, but Betty Gordon was gone.

Usually the women received their fluoroscope and pneumothorax treatment at separate times, but today there was some overlap because of the heavier surgery schedule and the increase in the number of patients, from both in and out of the sanatorium. The heavy schedule was noticeable. Doctor Sheridan's morning rounds were becoming more infrequent and the comforting feeling of the morning visits—an indication that he really cared—was missed. Doctor Herman was giving more pneumos now to both men and women. His internship would be completed in June and Doctor Sheridan was seeking a suitable replacement. With the military emergency there was a shortage of doctors. Even with the long hours, Doctor Harman was seeing more of Miss Sharen and Miss Downley. It was fascinating, great and wonderful. He was torn between two loves. Behavior at the hospital was most professional. Love was discernible only to each of the three lovers in its proper place.

Toward the end of March, at long last after much anxiety, Joe received a letter from Pat. As much as she wanted to see him, her parents wouldn't allow it and she was forbidden to write to him. The X-ray, which was taken at Good Samaritan Hospital, showed some signs of infection. The doctor had ordered three months of bed rest. Her parents would not permit her to go to a sanatorium and she had to spend three months resting at home. The days and nights were long and lonesome. Her next X-ray was scheduled in June and the doctor had said that she should be able to return to work then. It was wonderful to know that she would be all right. There was no serious infection and with proper rest and preventive measures she would be herself again, with all her cheerful, charming, graceful beauty. Reading her letter brightened his spirits with visions of the future when he would be well enough to walk outdoors. Spring was in the air. March roared out like a lion.

However, after another round of sputum checks, he was still positive. His spirits were dampened. With the arrival of the balmy breezes came the April showers.

Chapter IX

SHORTNESS OF BREATH

The dim light glowed yellow from the dial in the darkness and there was a humming sound above the fast excited voice of the news commentator. He could close his eyes and see his buddies there on Bataan as wave after wave of Japanese soldiers advanced. On a night such as this, April 11, 1942, Bataan surrendered after many a bloody charge was repelled. Often against regulations when he couldn't sleep, he would turn on his radio.

"Several of my buddies are on Bataan," he had said to Bunnigan one day when they were discussing the war.

Bunnigan, who wanted to get home to see his wife, had remarked in a sarcastic tone, "They ought to send guys like us to the front lines. We're no good to anyone here."

Randall had looked up from his Bible. "We wouldn't get to the front, much less fight."

"We could spray them with bugs," Skinner had chirped.

"Aha, ah-a. I get out of breath just taking my own bath," Towers had commented.

Darrell had wanted to enlist. He would never be able to enter the military service now. The war and the monotonous repetition of the commercial grated on his nerves, that sandpapery, itchy feeling that came with the commercial.

"...Do you have that itchy feeling in your throat? Try Dogan's cough medicine."

He turned off his radio disgustedly, then reached for a glass of water. He lit a cigarette, shielding the lighted match and squinting. Worried thoughts weighed heavily upon him. He had had three positive sputum checks. Why even after his adhesions were cut, and why, with all the pneumos, didn't he improve? And why had Doctor Sheridan warned him against fluid and empyema? Time was slowly slipping through his fingers. Would it ever end? He tried to tighten his grasp, but there was nothing, just the stillness of the night that always moved in only to be disturbed by the rattling snores, grinding teeth, and the occasional coughs. Miss Downley hadn't visited him in the past week. He was restless and irritable. Blood ran hot in his veins.

Several days ago his family had come to the sanatorium for their X-rays. They had come on different days. Seven little stairsteps, happy with laughter, had encircled his bed. He could see them now and he could hear their voices. The younger ones thought it was a joke. They couldn't understand why he was in bed.

"Why couldn't I have gone to the office to see them?" he had asked his dad when the children were gone.

"The doctor said that you aren't permitted up," Mr. Darrell had replied.

He had been infuriated. "Not permitted up! I go to the clinic every week for a pneumo and wait there sometimes more than an hour. It would seem that just this one time I could have gone to the office for a few minutes."

"The doctor said that it would be all right if they just stayed for a minute and the little ones wanted so much to see you, Joe," his mother had said.

"The risk is too great. I'd never forgive myself if this happened to them. The doctor wouldn't let his children come anywhere near the sanatorium," he had said. And in the quiet conversation that followed, he told his parents that three of Randall's sisters were here.

Mrs. Darrell had changed the subject. "The nurse told me that you had your adhesions cut, Joe."

He had unbuttoned the top of his pj's. The pink-blue scar was about an inch and a half long, and below the scar his side looked like a pin cushion without the pins, just the visible traces of white scar tissue that spotted his bony framework and one red scab.

"Looks as if you got hit with a load of buckshot," Mr. Darrell had commented.

A cough and a long drawn, rattling groan followed by a gurgling noise startled Darrell, who was half asleep with his thoughts. He sat up in bed. The fellow in the corner bed where he had once been, gave another gurgling groan. Other beds creaked and stirred in the darkness.

Towers had been transferred to the new building and Bunnigan had moved into the first bed; Darrell, into the fourth. Two commodes had been placed on each side of him, one for Skinner and the other for Dan Loness, who had the fifth bed.

No one spoke. Darrell reached for the button and gave it three quick flashes as Skinner turned on his bed lamp. He blinked and shuddered at the sight of blood, trickling from Dan's chin that stained and blotched the pillows.

Dan Loness was a harness race driver, a witty old codger, and he liked to hear Dan describe the sulky races. "Yeah," he had said, "getting a good start counted...time your horse and get her over on the rail as you turn to begin. Yes Sirree, I got my horse up there in a canter at the wave of the flag. They didn't cut out Ole Dan...no sirree, they had to get up early in the mornin' to beat Ole Dan..." He would extend his hard calloused hands as if he were holding the lines and the whip; his white hair, combed to one side, would flop across the side of his hawk nose and his bed was like a sulky to him when he waved his arms as if he were snapping the whip. "Crack the whip around their ears," Dan had said, "and she'll stretch her nose out there enough to win many a dead heat. Did you ever get over to the county fair, my boy? If you did, you saw me in the sulky races. I hit 'em all, my boy."

The nurse, Eve Stevens, appeared after what seemed to be an unusually long time. She wore a placid, yet sour, look as if she had been disturbed. She gave him a hypo and put an icepack on his chest. Shortly after the nurse left, Bunnigan entered carrying a book. When Eve Stevens was working nights, Bunnigan often tip-toed out of the room with a book under his arm. Until now, Darrell hadn't noticed that Bunnigan wasn't in his bed.

Darrell didn't remember falling asleep. Dan Loness, he thought, is driving his last race. The next morning when he awoke, Ole Dan had his head propped against the pillows. And that morning as usual, the curtains were drawn around the third and the fifth beds where the commodes stood. With the rising stench, he left the porch.

He returned saying, "I have a good high-classed name for this dump—Commodilly Row."

Bunnigan and Randall joined him in laughter as Skinner and Loness' faces grew red.

"I'm sure glad I've moved," bantered Bunnigan. "I can hardly wait to move to the new building."

That day Doc began pneumothorax treatment on Dan and he complained about the pressure that was in his chest. His wife came to visit him; she was a sweet, plump, little old lady, and in spite of Dan's saddened mood, she tried to cheer him with her laughter and stories about the races.

With the pneumothorax, Dan developed fluid and his temperature rose to 102. He tried to eat, but there was nothing that he was able to keep down and he grew weaker by the day. The loss of weight was noticeable; he seemed to melt away; his cheeks were drawn and his eyes had a glassy stare.

Occasionally, Transfusion talked to Dan. "I've had fluid for a couple of years now," he said as if to cheer him up, "and whenever I turn over in bed, I can hear it splash around in my side. Doc don't even bother to drain it off...Ha, he-a. I got a hole in my lung and I cough up the stuff. Ha, he-a...tastes awful, the green slimy stuff."

Once in awhile Dan would chuckle. However as the days passed, he grew weaker and weaker his face more drawn and gaunt, lying there with his eyes closed, wasting away. His wife could only look at him for a few minutes before she would break down with tears, but she came more often to see him and always spoke a few words with Darrell who had the bed next to him.

Darrell listened patiently as she talked of the good times that they had enjoyed together. She seemed to sense that Dan would not pull through and as Darrell watched him waste away, he feared, more than ever, the very thoughts of fluid and its effect. Even though he wasn't permitted to be up, he would occasionally join in the evening poker sessions. It was mainly to get away from his thoughts and the sight of Ole Dan who complained about his bedsores, for he lay on his back with little movement throughout the day and night.

Skinner was also playing poker; he had been raised to class one and a half, which permitted him to go to the bathroom once a day since his last sputum check was negative, as was Randall's. Uncomplainingly, Randall accepted his shortness of breath.

Often through the day and night while Randall was sitting up in bed, his head hung down and nodded with sleep that crept in upon him. Then he would awake with a jar as his arms gave way and his head hit the bed. Again he would straighten and brace himself until his arms gave way again with sleep. The fellows would stare at him not knowing what was happening or how to help him and they felt sorry for him.

"I ho-hope this phrenic doesn't last much longer," he would say. "I'm n-n-negative now, but I can't breathe."

Darrell was reminded of a statement often quoted by some of the patients at the sanatorium: "The operation was a success, but the patient died." And he could only sympathize with him.

One night, long after the lights were out, a booming crash hollowed across the porch. The fellows were jarred awake. There in the darkness upon the floor, Randall struggled and staggered as he arose and climbed back into bed. That morning Darrell told Miss Sharen what had happened and asked her to see if anything could be done to help Randall.

"Why do you sit up in bed?" queried Doctor Sheridan when he was making his morning rounds.

"I get-get so short of breath. Th-that's the only way I can catch my br-breath."

"Have you tried to sleep with your bed raised?"

"It-it doesn't help."

The doctor considered putting side boards on his bed, but Randall told him that he would bump his head on the boards when he fell asleep.

"We'll put you in a low bed," said the doctor with a glance toward Miss Boswell and Miss Sharen who had accompanied him.

On the first of every month, as a matter of record, the patients were weighed. Darrell had gained about ten pounds. His weight was 160, and his pleural wall had toughened, and more pressure was applied as the needle jabbed and pierced its way through the protective wall. At intervals of five days, he received pneumos, a dreaded experience, which forced the infected portion of his lung to collapse giving his body a chance to fight the invading bugs or to seal them into a calcareous tomb. The little termites in their waxy covered shells withstood all known germs produced by medical science. Literature circulated through the ward about these invading termites, but he could read very little of it. The sight of the destruction caused by them left him despondent. He preferred to read historical novels. The sanatorium contained a small library, which had been donated and maintained by a local women's club. The librarian was a former patient who volunteered her services. Each week she made her rounds of the patients with a small selection of books on a library cart. She was helpful and her visits were most welcomed. She helped Skinner select books that were on the required reading list for high school students. Randall's reading was limited now to his Bible. Bunnigan was an avid reader who also liked to read historical novels.

When Mother's Day arrived, Mrs. Skinner placed a large bouquet of lilacs on the dresser by the windows and stepped back to admire them. The breeze that blew in through the open windows was balmy and sweetened by the fragrance of the pink-purple lilacs that reflected in the mirror on the brick wall behind them.

Paul Skinner turned up his nose. "Flowers always remind me of funerals."

"Why Paul, the flowers are beautiful and have a nice fragrance and will improve your attitude. Some of the other fellows might like them," said Mrs. Skinner as Mr. Skinner who was seated in the metal lounge chair, rocked back and forth as usual.

Bunnigan, who had obtained permission for this special day, was leaving the room to go riding with his wife, when Joe's brother Charles and his sisters, Mary, Ruth and Norma entered. The awkwardness of the first several visits had worn away and their talk was more relaxed. He listened eagerly as they talked of the results of their recent X-rays.

"Bernadette's X-ray was a blank," said Mary, laughingly. "We told her not to move, but she wiggled, squirmed and laughed. Daddy's X-ray was good, not even a scar. I guess all the work in the fresh air keeps him healthy."

"I have a small scar," said Charles, "but it's healed. I'm A-1 and ready for the army. I expect to get my greetings one of these days."

"How about your X-ray?"

"It's fine," Norma replied.

Mary and Ruth answered likewise.

"But," continued Mary, "Madonna and Richard will have to come back for another X-ray in three months."

Idle chatter followed. Nothing was said about Mother's X-ray. He took it for granted that it was all right. The thought never occurred to him that anything could be wrong.

Mary took a step forward, admiring the lilacs. "Remember the two big bushes of white and purple lilacs that we had when we lived at Dayton? You'd cut a big bouquet for Mother every Mother's Day."

"Yes, and then we'd sell as many of the cut lilacs as we could to the neighbors. What the neighbors didn't buy I would sell door to door. The few dollars that we made was an extra present for both Mother and Dad."

"You remember how we use to raid the neighbor's cherry orchard?" asked Charles.

"Yeah," Joe replied with a chuckle. "We ate until we were ready to burst. You were supposed to keep a lookout. I looked down and spotted Farmer Bowman sneaking toward us. When I yelled, you jumped and ran for the cornfields, and I fell when I jumped. He was right on top of me...well, almost...he took after me and you branched the other way."

Charles laughed. "Yeah, that was funny. You always could run faster than I. I could see the top of him from the waist up, but I couldn't see you."

"He was faster than I. I couldn't get away from him on the straight-a-way, so I cut through the rows of drilled corn. He almost had me when he stumbled."

Their idle chatter continued as they told of tricks that were played on each other. He forgot about his mother's X-ray and the fact that he was still positive. It was a joyful visit and it helped him to feel better.

By the next bed where Ole Dan lay, his wife and their sons and daughter were gathered around, looking very solemn and grieved. More relatives and neighbors came. Some of them began to cry.

Joe's brother and sisters left, saddened by the gathering at the next bed, and he was alone. The low sobs from the relatives gathered around Dan's bed made him feel very sorry for Dan, and he dreaded the thoughts of fluid and the effects it had on Dan. Ole Dan was a bundle of bones. He hardly realized what was going on around him. He wanted to be moved to a private room, as did his family, but there were none available.

When Mr. and Mrs. Randall entered, stares of amazement encompassed them. For a while they talked softly to Gene. Then Mr. Randall walked around the foot of the low bed nervously wringing his hands, his huge frame moved in a slow deliberate motion as he paced over to the bouquet of lilacs that stood on the dresser. Momentarily, he gazed at the flowers, then paced back to the side of his wife. They stood there with their heads drooped, looking down upon Gene. One leg was crossed before him and the other dangled over the side with his toes touching the floor as he struggled for breath.

It was indeed a sad Mother's Day and he thought it was strange that his mother hadn't come to visit him. It had been several weeks since he had last seen her, however he thought that at this time of the year there was always an endless amount of work on the farm. Dad was very busy in the fields getting out the spring crops and Mother never finished her work, the cooking, the cleaning, and the sewing. Now, with school almost over, there were always so many extra duties with at least seven in school and Norma was graduating from high school this year. His thoughts drifted to his graduation...the class play...the Junior-Senior Prom...the class day out along the lake...and his valedictorian speech at the Alumni Banquet... "We who stand between a happy past and an unknown future, it seems well for us to consider what our future is or ought to be as citizens of a great Republic—the greatest in all the world..." He had heard of several athletic scholarship offers in basketball, but neither he nor his parents could afford the other expenses.

Weeks passed and there was no word from home. He had received a negative sputum check and he had written a letter to Pat. He described the classes from one to twelve, and as he calculated the time required for each, he informed her that he hoped to be released in another year. But now that he was negative, maybe her doctor and parents would permit her to visit him. He had visions of being raised to class two and he anxiously awaited word from her.

After four negative checks and a negative culture, Bunnigan was raised to class two. His infection was not as advanced as that of the others on the sunporch and his phrenic was apparently effective. The progress was encouraging, but Bunnigan was also a diabetic. Medical research was also making some progress. In 1940, F. Bernheim had found that benzoic and salicylic acids promoted the metabolism of tubercle bacilli and he suggested that other derivatives might have a reverse effect. It appeared to be the beginning of research in the right direction after many years of basic research. A Swedish investigator, J. Lehmann found that one of these derivatives, para-aminosalicylic acid (PAS), inhibited the growth and multiplication of tubercle bacilli. It would be years before it could be made available for clinical use. For many of the patients, the results of many long years of research, investigation, testing and tireless effort would not come soon enough. Artificial pneumothorax was the most widely used treatment. For some where pneumothorax failed or could not be used, a new type of chest surgery became necessary—a reduction in the rib cage by the removal of some of the ribs (thoracoplasty). Doctor Sheridan had performed a number of thoracoplasty surgeries here. He was participating in the development and introduction of excisional surgery techniques for the removal of single lobes of the lungs, and he was trying to arrange for the extended training of Doctor Harman who was his assistant. Much of the training, study, investigation, testing, development and research were disrupted by the military emergency at that time. The discovery of many early lesions during the induction screening made the need for knowing how to handle those more urgent.

The first week of June came and went. Lying in bed became more tiresome and monotonous for Darrell. His father made an unexpected visit. He had left Doctor Sheridan's office and was standing by his bedside where he talked in a very quiet voice.

Joe's eyes flashed and opened wide with surprise. "What did Doctor Sheridan say?"

"That Mother's last X-ray showed some signs of change from the previous one that was taken three months ago and that Mother needs rest and quiet," said his father in low, solemn, almost lost tones of voice, and he shook his head in silence.

As if to offer some encouragement, Joe said, "I've read in some of the literature and reports that some of the changes appearing in X-rays are limited by some changes in the lungs and by the difficulty of differentiating these changes due to other conditions. The X-ray will hopefully appear much better with the next one."

"I can't understand it. Mother never coughs, has no fever, and has never had any of the symptoms. She looks as healthy as ever."

"Perhaps Mother could have an examination and an X-ray somewhere else."

"We can't change it and we can't afford any added expense. Mary and Charles are working and helping out, but this is too much." There was a pause. His father's lips began to quiver with the thoughts of losing her. "It's going to be awful for the children for Mother to be here," said his father, and with slowly moistening eyes, he left the sunporch.

He didn't know what to do. He felt as if he were to blame, but he had to accept it and hope for the best.

Chapter X

DARRELL'S MOTHER IS ADMITTED

The days were hot and sultry with the approaching summer. The sanatorium residents were lost in the daily routine that never ended. Joe, sad to say, awaited the arrival of his mother and on the lawn below the windows, the fellows played croquet. Actually the fellows from the new building who were in the higher classes were permitted outdoor exercise. They were all laughing and having a grand time. Several of the nurses stopped for a few minutes. Among them was Mary Jane Downley. The sun reflected the gold in her light brown hair and under the brilliant solar rays, the beauty of her form was comparable to the Venus de Milo.

A wheelchair was shoved into the open doorway and Mrs. Darrell arose slowly and walked toward Joe's bed. She was wearing a new, dusty-pink chenille robe; one that Mary, Eileen and Norma had given to her for this occasion. There was a smile upon the fullness of her cheeks.

"I hate to come through the men's ward looking this way," she said as she seated herself in the folding chair by his bed. "It's much too hot and uncomfortable to wear a corset."

He smiled as best he could, but the fact that his mother was here, like this, was heartbreaking. How could he ever be forgiven?

"There will be another little one in the family," she remarked. There was a pause. He could tell that she was pregnant. Fifteen children...and what if the baby were born here at the sanatorium? Perhaps that was the reason for the change in the appearance of her X-ray.

"What did the doctor say about your X-ray?" he asked at length.

"That I have a clouded area on my lungs. The county health doctor made such a fuss. He said that I would infect the children and he even threatened to take them away if I wouldn't consent to come here. I never cough or raise anything from my lungs. I can't understand it."

"You must see another doctor. You certainly look as healthy as ever. It's difficult to believe there is anything wrong," said Joe, encouragingly.

His mother returned the compliment. "You're looking much better and you have gained some weight."

"My last sputum check was negative, but according to my last X-ray, the doctor said that the infiltration on my left lung wasn't clearing as it should." He paused, then added, "Who's taking care of the children?"

"Norma," she answered. "But Daddy is so upset. He has so much to do. I'm worried. I don't know how he's going to take all of this."

An emotional pause followed. A nurse entered with the wheelchair.

"I must go now. The nurse is waiting to take me back."

"Maybe I can get permission to visit you, Mother."

"Yes, because I hate to come through the wards this way. Since my pregnancy is so pronounced, it always shows so much more on me," she added as she arose to leave.

Bunnigan, Skinner, and Randall were shocked and asked many questions about his mother. He answered their questions quietly. They couldn't understand it either. She looked so healthy. They added sympathizing comments in a cheery manner.

They were still talking, very quietly, when Ole Dan raised his bones and began to yell with a sudden spurt of life.

"Get up in there you old son of a gun!" he shouted in a hollow cry, waving his bony arm as if he were cracking the whip. "Get the lead out of your ass!"

Miss Sharen, who was on duty at the time, heard him yell and rushed in to see what the commotion was about. When she saw him, her steps slowed and her face stiffened.

He didn't see her or much of anything else, and another hollow cry echoed much shriller. "Get the lead out!"

The fellows, at first very much amazed, laughed amusedly in spite of the spectacle. They laughed more at Miss Sharen who paused momentarily.

"Mr. Loness," she said sternly.

He crumpled, gasping short and fast for breath.

Later he was transferred to one of the small cubbyholes that served as a dingy private room. Large double doors opened from the sunporch into the four cubbyholes. These doors remained closed now since the porch had been converted into a ward of five beds, except when the patients roamed through them as Transfusion did.

Bob Robbins was transferred into the fifth bed in the far corner. He was one of the old lungers, though only twenty-four years of age. He talked in a breathy voice that emphasized his light complexion and his straight blonde hair as he related his experiences of the last six years, most of which were spent in this sanatorium.

"I spent more than three years on my first cure," said

Robbins, "or rather, an apparent cure. Old Doctor Blare was in charge then."

Skinner was laughing and interrupted. "He use to give 1000 cc's of air at a crack, and he'd throw that needle like a dart."

"He...he didn't believe in surgery," added Randall from his sitting position in the low bed. "With 1000 cc's of air, B-Blare tried to snap any ad-adhesions."

"When I was released," continued Robbins, "I took a bus to join my dad in Northern California where he lived at that time. The first several days of my trip were fine, but on the third day I couldn't eat and when I arrived in California, Dad took me to a hospital. There my sputum was positive and the doctor told Dad that from the looks of my X-ray, my cavity had never been closed or healed. Dad couldn't afford to keep me there and when I arrived here again, I was coughing blood. Doc Blare said it was just one of those things—some make it, and some don't. I helped to improve his record for releases, but the record for breakdowns was increased. I was so mad I couldn't see. So what happens? Just because of Blare, I'm all messed up. Doctor Sheridan wanted to give me thoracoplasty, but I wouldn't have him cutting my ribs out. So then he gave me a paraffin pack."

"What's that?" asked Darrell.

Robbins took off the top of his pajamas and showed the scar on his back where part of a rib had been removed and paraffin packed into its place to collapse the infected area of the lung.

"After a period of time," said Robbins, "the paraffin is absorbed, and by that time the lung should be healed. It has helped," he added. "I'm negative now, and I didn't want the scars and crushed chest that go with thoracoplasty for the rest of my life."

Skinner and Randall looked dubious; as a rule paraffin packs weren't too successful. Robbins reached for his light to drive away the sinister shadows of dusk that were creeping in upon the sunporch with the smell of death. In the corridor, voices and footsteps of nurses hurried about and the low rumble of a stretcher was heard passing through the shadows.

Transfusion swayed onto the porch into the yellow glow of Robbins' bed lamp, then stopped by the open windows, peering into the murky vastness. The low faint whistle of a slow freight could be heard in the distance.

"Ole Dan didn't make a sound," he said, still peering into the darkness.

"You mean he's..." Darrell paused. The thought of death had never occurred to him until now, although there had been other deaths.

"Yep, he kicked off," said Transfusion. "No one knew it until the night nurse came around. What a surprise it was to her. She asked him two times if he wanted any chocolate milk."

"Ran his last race. He was a real likable old codger," added Darrell.

There was another long low whistle from the freight train, fainter than before.

"What I wouldn't give to be riding the rods tonight," said Transfusion with a chuckle.

"I'm with you," injected Darrell. He had been sitting up in bed and the cold damp air from the window forced him to lie back and pull up a blanket.

"I've rode 'em in every state of the Union." Transfusion chuckled again and licked his chops. "Use to cook stew in the jungles with the boys—everybody was welcome and it all went in one pot...Ho, ho-o."

When Darrell laughed, a sharp pain stabbed like a knife from the right side across his chest.

"I got time for one game," said Bunnigan, who had been visiting some of the patients down the hall.

"Aren't you gonna play, Darrell?" asked Skinner, getting out of bed.

"I don't know. I think I've got pleurisy," he replied, wincing as another sharp pain shot across to his heart.

"You guys get a pain and you think you gonna die," taunted Bunnigan as he turned on the overhead lights.

"If you've got pleurisy," remarked Transfusion, "about all you can do for it is to keep your side warm." Then he opened his robe and pulled up the back of his pajamas. "See that? I wear this red woolen band to keep my side warm. My pleurisy comes and goes. It has for years."

He stared at his bony ribs and the red band. Damn! Is there anything that this guy doesn't have? he wondered.

"Pleurisy is a bad sign," commented Robbins, getting up to play poker.

"Why?" queried Darrell.

"That's how my fluid started," commented Transfusion, "but that doesn't mean that you'll have fluid."

"If we re gonna play, we'd better get started. It's after eight," remarked Bunnigan.

Joe remained in bed nursing his side as the fellows gathered around the card table, and he remembered that the pressure readings, while he had received his last three pneumos, had changed from a negative to a positive reading.

Skinner reared back in his chair and squealed like a stuck hog. "Sandbagging huh? Sit back and check the nuts to me."

Bunnigan roared with laughter. " I only want to teach you not to be so cocksure."

Skinner's face grew red and in his mind he was figuring a way to even the score.

Joe's laughter was cut short by another sharp pain.

When Doctor Sheridan made his rounds the following morning, he had intended to tell him, however the pain wasn't as sharp and besides, he wanted to obtain permission to see his mother.

"May I visit Mother today?" he asked.

"I would much rather have your mother visit you," answered the doctor, then added, "Furthermore, I wouldn't like to have you roam through the women's ward."

He had hoped to visit Betty Gordon also. He started to suggest a possible alternative, but his words were drowned by the laughter of the doctor and the fellows as the doctor proceeded out the door, followed by Miss Boswell who joined in the laughter.

Mary, Ruth, and Norma stopped to visit him that afternoon after seeing Mother. In spite of everything, they appeared very jolly.

"Look what we bought for you when we were shopping!" said Mary.

"And here's a carton of cigarettes," added Ruth, before he could reply.

"Mother said you should stop smoking," said Norma.

"I am cutting down on the cigarettes; only a half a pack a day now," he said and his eyes lit up. He was as pleased as a kid with a new toy. "This is a little tiny horse!"

"You always did like horses," said Mary. "And don't give this little cactus too much water."

On his bed stand, he placed the tiny, cream-colored china horse with the potted cactus upon its back, and thanking Ruth, he placed the cigarettes in the drawer.

"Have you heard from Pat?" asked Norma.

"I received a letter. Her parents will not permit her to visit me."

Mary changed the subject. "We tried to find a billy goat. Remember the day you came home from school with a big white billy goat?"

He laughed. "How could I forget. One of the boys in my class, Raymond Tindell, couldn't keep the goat any longer and said his father told him that he had to get rid of the goat or he would kill it. I was in the sixth grade then."

"We were living on Old Troy Pike in the outskirts of Dayton," continued Mary. "And when you got home with the goat, he was bigger than you. Uncle Herman was talking to Mother by the banister of the porch." Mary burst into laughter as she continued, "The old billy goat started to baa-a and reared straight up on its hind legs, then made a dash for him. Uncle Herman jumped over the banister, knocking Mother's flower pots to the ground and the goat started to eat the flowers."

He was laughing so much that tears came to his eyes.

"That old goat with his long horns," continued Mary with laughter, "...how the kids ran; they were scared stiff."

He interrupted. "We had a lot of fun with that old billy goat. A year later when we were moving from Dayton to Celina, the goat was in the back of our old open pickup and whenever we'd stop for traffic, the goat would baa-a and baa-a. The people would laugh their heads off. What a sight we were—the pickup piled high with furniture and a big white billy goat."

When the laughter had ceased, Mary changed the conversation.

"Mother was looking good."

"She would like to see you," said Norma.

"So would I, but Doc said that he'd rather have Mother visit me. He doesn't want me to visit the women's ward and keeps telling me to stay in bed. I'll keep asking him and maybe he'll give me permission."

After a few comments that followed, his sisters left. That evening the sharp jabbing pain seemed to penetrate even deeper with each breath he took and his breathing became very shallow. When he awoke the following morning, he felt feverish. His pajamas were soggy with cold perspiration that had a soured scent. He examined his thermometer closely. It read 102.

Chapter XI

DARRELL DEVELOPS EMPYEMA

On the first day of July, the slanted rays of the sun cast a darkened shadow as a black hearse rolled lazily over the lonesome, winding drive that encircled the well-kept lawn to the rear of the ivy-walled sanatorium. The fellows on the sunporch, with the exception of Darrell, watched with downcast eyes as the hearse crawled to a stop at the elevator entrance directly below the windows and then spoke banteringly.

"He made the sure cure," commented Skinner.

"Yep, there he goes, toes up!" added Transfusion as if he could see through the white sheet that was draped across the stretcher.

"The majority of 'em die in bed," added Bunnigan. "Ole Dan never left his bed. He took a good cure."

"His heart stopped," said Randall who remained there staring, his face expressionless as he struggled for breath.

In the fourth bed, Darrell, who was burning with a 102 fever, listened to their depressing conversation. With each breath that he took, the pain in his chest had cut like a knife throughout that day. It continued on into the next, and the next, day after day. Each bite of food swelled with the nauseated acids that well-up within until they gripped his throat. The milk that he drank only churned in his stomach, forcing him to leave the bed for the bathroom in spite of his weakness. Each meal of the day was the same procedure, again and again. The trays of food were sent back almost the same as he had received them, and he could hear the grumblings from the lady in charge of the food conveyor. Then Miss Sharen suggested a diet of soft foods and after speaking to the doctor, she was able to get a special tray for him. Even the soft foods he wasn't able to keep down. However, he managed to sip the broth and keep it down. The fellows shook their heads saying, "You've got to eat. You can't live without eating." He watched with chagrin as the fellows around him ate the good solid foods that he had liked so well. His laughter was gone, but there was a feeble grin the night that Skinner shoved his tray aside.

"Look at these hamburger balls," Skinner said with disdain.

"Who could eat this stuff?" Then he bounced one off the brick wall and caught it on the rebound. "If that chef were here, I'd bounce one off his noggin."

Transfusion ambled aimlessly onto the porch. "How did you guys like the rubber-burgers?"

"They make good rubber bumpers. Would you like one?" asked Skinner.

"I couldn't eat the ones I had," chuckled Transfusion and added, "Darrell, you can feel lucky that you didn't get any."

"The hamburger looked good to me. How lucky you are to be able to eat solid food."

But Darrell felt anything but lucky. Although, Miss Sharen was kind and considerate and did everything possible to make him more comfortable. She pounded and straightened the pillows and added words of encouragement while she rubbed his back with alcohol and patted on the powder, telling him not to lie in one position.

That week Miss Downley relieved Miss Sharen on her day off, but Darrell was much too sick to appreciate her care, the bed bath, or the back rub, and when she added fruit juice to his diet, the lady in charge of the food conveyor grumbled in protest and refused without a doctor's approval.

"You'd think that she was paying for it," said Darrell. "Who is she?"

"Her husband is the controller," replied Robbins from the bed next to Darrell.

"They have a real set-up," added Bunnigan. "He practically runs this place.

"What's his name?" asked Darrell.

"You've seen him," continued Bunnigan. "Mr. Beetle, a short, slender built, red-faced guy with beady eyes."

"Oh yes, he looks like a weasel," said Darrell. "Beetle stood by the door the day the commissioners came around. He always points out the fat rosy-cheeked patients who are flushed with fever, but the commissioners don't know it."

"That's the one day of the month that the chef puts out a real good meal," said Robbins, and the fellows burst into laughter.

"You can always tell when the commissioners have a meeting here," added Bunnigan.

Before Miss Downley went off duty that day she said, "Mr. Darrell, promise me that you will eat better." And taking a step nearer she added, "I'll talk to Doctor Sheridan about the fruit juice and perhaps you should also."

He was captivated by the sincerity of her voice and the enchanting smile upon her lips. Momentarily, he forgot that nauseated feeling that was always present.

"I like to see you smile," she said.

There was a pause when neither spoke as their eyes met and lingered there, yearning for something that could not be.

He was standing by the card table the following morning

when Doctor Sheridan entered the room earlier than usual. He was waiting while Miss Sharen made up his bed.

The doctor spoke in a voice that was very quiet. "You better sit down before you fall down."

He seated himself; his face was very pale. That isn't very encouraging. It's not like Doctor Sheridan at all, he thought.

Still speaking in a quiet voice, the doctor added, "I'll fluoroscope you tomorrow and see how much fluid you have."

"Could you have fruit juices added to my diet? I'm not able to eat much of anything."

"You're on a soft diet, aren't you?"

"All I'm able to keep down is the broth."

"What about milk?"

Darrell shook his head. "When I try to drink milk, I lose the broth."

"All right, I'll speak to the dietitian."

The following morning, Darrell was seated on the stretcher at the clinic. Doctor Sheridan stood before him, jabbed a needle between his ribs, attached a small syringe that drew off 50 cc's of fluid at a time, and squirted it into a basin that the nurse held.

"That's a nasty color," he said.

The greenish-yellow liquid was indeed sickening to see and he gripped the edge of the stretcher, afraid of falling. He could feel the pull of the syringe as it was filled over and over again until there was a gurgling sound within his chest.

"That sounds like the last of it," said Sheridan, and added as if it might be some consolation, "That was 800 cc's. You had plenty."

Then he was wheeled to his bed. The pleurisy in his right side continued, though not as severe. However, his temperature remained at 102 and with it, there was that qualmishness and that soured perspiration with the stale putrid scent. If this fluid was nature's way to fight the infection, he hoped that it wouldn't last too long. In keeping with his promise to Miss Downley, he sipped all the broth and found the orange juice to be refreshing. He even managed to drink some of the milk. Mrs. Beetle, the lady at the food conveyor, grumbled every time she served a glass of juice. Occasionally, she would raise her voice for Darrell's benefit.

"Here, this is for that demanding baby on the sunporch."

Skinner mimicked her in a high-pitched voice, "Demanding baby. I heard what you said!"

Transfusion wobbled onto the porch chuckling. "What did you do to the Queen of the Pots?"

"Beats me, but it must be killing her to serve a bowl of broth and a glass of orange juice," said Darrell.

She was furious, and Miss Sharen had to reprimand Skinner to calm her.

In the days that followed, Mrs. Beetle continued to grumble. Darrell was too weary to care, and it was through Miss Sharen's care and influence that he continued to receive the various fruit juices. His side was aspirated again. There were 100 cc's of purulent fluid, a yellowish-white matter. He trembled at the sight of it and there was a look of astonishment, or perhaps more of grief or uneasiness, on the doctor's face.

"Some Azocloramid solution," Doctor Sheridan said to the nurse.

Darrell's pleural cavity was irrigated with the cold solution. He felt very low, as depressed as he thought he could be. For the past two weeks, the fluid and the high fever had killed his desire to see his mother. Only a few notes had been exchanged and he didn't tell her how sick he really was. His dad came every Sunday now, since his mother was here, and Joe had tried to appear as cheerful as he could. His temperature hovered around 102. The loss of weight was noticeable. He feared the thoughts of lying helplessly in bed as Dan had done, and he made a real effort to get out of bed and walk to the bathroom and back, at least twice a day, morning and evening. Occasionally, some of the fellows from the new building had come to visit him. Bill Read, who was from Darrell's home town, had visited him frequently. Today, shortly after Darrell had been returned to his bed, Towers and Bill Read stopped on the sunporch.

"Okay you guys, get up out of bed!" said Read. "We've just come from the office and Doc's got a cure. Just a shot of this stuff in the arm is all you need."

The fellows stared wide-eyed. Even Randall, who was half-asleep, raised his head in amazement. They had followed the advances of medical science and hailed the discoveries of the new sulfa drugs and the development of penicillin. Medical science, they thought, had done it at last.

"You guys can start packing your bags," said Towers, "and go through the office with your sleeves rolled up."

"Medical science hasn't begun," said Bunnigan. "This is 1942, and for the most part there has been no effective medical research or discoveries made in the TB field since the use of the X-ray around 1895."

"Has it been a question of financial resources? Was the sale of Christmas Seals sufficient?" asked Darrell. "Evidentially not. But look at the amount of money that is being spent on the war effort and all the foreign aid programs. Would a charge of five or ten dollars per person a year for research and preventive measures be worth it?" There was no immediate response and Darrell continued, "Had we had a program of that magnitude, maybe we wouldn't be here."

"In 1940 came the Draft Act and a requirement to screen all eligible persons for TB," said Bunnigan. The same requirement was imposed before in 1917 for screening the manpower prior to induction into military service during World War I. We may see the day when we have better control and enforcement of screening for the general public."

"If so, the public wouldn't be exposed as we were," said Darrell.

"It was a nice dream. Anyway you guys look like you need a shot in the arm," said Read looking around the room.

"I'm afraid it's to-too late for me," said Randall, shaking his head and trying to catch his breath.

"It's never too late. And it's a good thought; makes me feel better," said Darrell.

"How's the fluid?" asked Towers.

Darrell shook his head. "Doc irrigated my side this morning. I've got empyema now."

There was a pause before Towers commented encouragingly,

"That might help to get rid of some of the infection."

"What class are you in, Towers?"

"Class eight. I'm taking my half hour of walking exercise."

"And you, Bill?"

"Class twelve; means three hours of walking."

"You'll be leaving soon."

"I was only raised to twelve yesterday, which means about three more months for me. I'm one of the old lungers, not as fortunate as these military draftees whose infection isn't as serious or advanced. I spent more than two and a half years here."

"Bunnigan, when are you moving to the new building?" asked Towers.

"I've been in class two for six weeks," replied Bunnigan, "but Doc wants me to wait awhile because I just have a phrenic, and if that doesn't work or help to keep my lung at rest on my left side, it means thoracoplasty, or so he says."

When Read and Towers had gone, Darrell felt somewhat better after their discussion or dreams of the development of improved controls and techniques for detecting TB and chemotherapy. "A shot in the arm," as Read had called it. But it was a struggle to maintain enough strength to go to the bathroom.

He would stare at his face in the bathroom mirror and see, reflected there, a pallid, languid expression. A third week of fluid passed and his side was aspirated for the third time. He was seated on the stretcher and Doctor Harman stood beside him as Doctor Sheridan jabbed the needle between the usual ribs. A sharp pain shot to his shoulder, almost jerking him off the stretcher. His arm flew up and his head jerked.

"Oh! I struck your diaphragm."

The room began to whirl and a nauseating acid filled his throat. His face was as white as the sheet on the stretcher.

"Feel weak?" asked Doctor Harman who was holding him.

The room stopped spinning. "I'm all right now," he said.

"Tell me when I stick your diaphragm," said Doctor Sheridan, ready to jab the needle a rib higher.

It all happened so fast, Darrell wondered how he could tell him. With the next jab, the needle missed his diaphragm and also missed the pocket of fluid. He was jabbed again on a downward angle, more to the right.

"His diaphragm is creeping up along his pleural wall," said Sheridan to Harman.

Brilliant deduction, thought Darrell.

The needle had revived Darrell with each jab, but a faintness seized him as the syringe drew the purulent fluid into its vacuum.

"Eighty cc's," said Sheridan to the nurse who entered the amount on his file records.

Then there was the cold gurgling sensation as his pleural cavity was irrigated with the Azocloramid solution, again and again, before air was added to hold the upper lobe as his lung collapsed. Mary Boswell, the superintendent of nurses, who helped occasionally when more critical attention was required and because of the shortage of trained nurses, wheeled him to the sunporch.

As he stepped from the chair, the fellows and the beds reeled with dizziness before him. Each foot reached out blindly and limply—he staggered, then dropped away. The nurse gripped him about the shoulders and struggled him to his bed where he fell across it. The room reeled clear with whiffs of ammonia. The nurse, leaning over him, wiped the beads of cold perspiration from his forehead with a cool cloth and added a smile of kindness. She returned a few minutes later and handed him a letter that had arrived in the morning mail, as if she knew that it was a special letter. It was from Pat. She had planned to visit him, but as expected, her parents wouldn't permit it. Her doctor had informed her that her last X-ray was much better. After three months of rest, she was working part-time on assignment for special exhibits and expected to be working full-time soon. She planned to visit sometime. He wondered if he would ever see her again. He was weak, exhausted and so wretched. As much as he wanted to see her radiant smile and beauty, to hear her cheerful, charming voice that was always so full of life, and to feel the touch of her hand once again, she was so far away. He was heartbroken.

The following morning, after a miserable sleep, he awoke earlier than usual. He shuffled to the bathroom, looked with a fixed gaze at his sad, sallow face, ran his fingers through his hair, and stared at his hand. His hair was falling by the handful. Slowly, he trudged back to his bed and buried his face in the pillows. Would it ever end, this lasting fever? Another day of the same routine—the broth, the orange juice, and the milk. Day after day, week after week, the same weary routine. And the days and nights continued hot and muggy. There was no air conditioning in the old sanatorium, only the wide open windows.

Chapter XII

A NEW NURSE REPLACES MISS DOWNLEY

August finally came. Doctor Herman had left for his assignment at a Toronto, Canada hospital and a continuation of his surgical training. The patients missed him and Doctor Sheridan, needless to say, was busier than ever. A higher percentage of the new patients were the more fortunate ones, thanks to the improvements in X-ray techniques and equipment and most of all to the screening done by the armed forces to protect all personnel. This was a form of preventive care that was seldom used or practiced until now, except in the national emergencies of World War I and II. Youth, with all its ambitions and exposure, had suffered the consequences.

With the coming of August, another weigh day arrived. Darrell had lost nineteen pounds in the past month.

"One hundred and forty," announced Miss Sharen as he stepped off the scales. "When I come back, I want to see you eating again."

"Are you going anywhere special?"

"Toronto, for a two week vacation."

He would miss her. Her patience and thoughtful care had

been wonderful. She had gone beyond her normal duty to obtain a soft diet and orange juice for him. "It will be cooler there. Are you from Toronto?"

"No, just visiting friends," she said and added, "There will be a new nurse starting on this floor tomorrow."

There was a look of disappointment on his face. He had hoped that Miss Downley would take her place while she was on vacation.

"Don't look so downhearted," she added as Darrell climbed into bed, "I'll be back."

There had been a drop in his fever that morning and what a pleasant feeling it was. His spirits had risen and there was a lightness about him as his smile returned. When Doctor Sheridan accompanied by Mary Boswell were making their rounds that morning, he asked for permission to visit his mother.

The doctor shook his head thoughtfully. "Do you feel that you're able?"

His face brightened. "My temperature was down this morning and I feel much better."

The doctor continued to shake his head. "What was it?"

"100.2," he replied, and a slight smile crossed his face.

There was a pause while the doctor contemplated; his face showed a release of tension. It was an unexpected, marvelous improvement, which occurred sooner than he had anticipated. Miss Boswell showed the doctor his chart. "I'll have the nurse wheel you over this evening for a short visit."

He managed to eat all the soft foods that were served to him that day; the first full meals in more than a month. Miss Sharen was working split hours and when she went off duty at seven, she wheeled him through the corridor to the elevator. There they rode to the first floor, then through the much narrower and dim corridors that separated the men's wards from the women's ward which was located in the eastern half. She was excited about her coming vacation and as the corridors widen, she began to push him faster, joking, laughing and commenting on her vacation that was soon to begin. When they passed the rooms, some of the women raised their heads slightly while others who were walking about in their rooms, stopped to stare wide-eyed, while others lay deathly still. There were women in a sorry condition. At the southeast corner of the corridor, Miss Sharen opened the door to the sunroom.

"Mrs. Darrell, look who came to see you," she said as she wheeled him into the room alongside his mother's bed.

"I heard he was very sick," she replied, smiling gracefully to the nurse and then to her son.

Four women, all about Mrs. Darrell's age, occupied the square room. There were two beds along the south and east walls in the adjacent corners. Opposite them along the inner wall facing south, were two more beds. The one nearer the door was Mrs. Darrell's.

The nurse held the door momentarily while she smiled down at him, then glancing to his mother she said, "He's feeling much better and he's beginning to eat again."

"She's a nice nurse," commented Mrs. Darrell when the door had closed.

"Yes, her care has meant a great deal to me," he said thoughtfully. "I'll miss her when she goes on her vacation tomorrow. She was instrumental in adding broth to my diet when I couldn't eat anything."

After his mother had introduced the other women, she showed him the doilies that she had made. There were three to a set, made with cream and red wine-colored cord. She explained how they were made on the tatting frame.

"That would be something for you to do, Joe."

He gave a little laugh showing not the least bit of interest.

"What class are you in?" he asked.

"I don't know," she replied. "I'm allowed to go to the bathroom, but I'm not permitted to take my own bath and those bed baths are terrible."

He chuckled as he thought of his first bed bath. "You must be in class two."

"I was supposed to send in a sputum specimen, but I can't raise anything, never have. The women say that I have no business being here."

"I don't think so either. You need to get another X-ray and another medical opinion."

"The women say that I'll help to improve the records—a patient released and sent home cured." She paused as she nodded her head toward the bed in the corner to the right. "Mrs. Tice, the thin women, has two boys, one three and the other seven. She had thoracoplasty about six months ago with nine ribs taken out on one side." Mrs. Darrell shook her head. "She has been here almost two years. The doctor raised her to class two this morning. And there's Mrs. Willowby with the snow-white hair in the other corner. She has been here three years. She said her hair turned white from being here. She won't let the doctor take any of her ribs out and she complains about everything: the doctors, the nurses, the food, the weather, and her aches and pains. Mrs. Biddle in the next bed is always smiling and joking. She showed me how to make the doilies. She gets pneumos on both lungs and has for more than a year. It's a pity. I don't know how she can stand it, but I guess we learn to live with it after awhile. Her eyes bother her and she was so surprised to learn that I had only one eye. I usually take out my glass eye at night."

Joe pointed toward the east windows. "There goes Doctor Sheridan with his pony and one of the little girls."

"Mrs. Willowby says he thinks more of that pony than he does of her." Mrs. Darrell was shaking her head and a slight smile crossed her face. "I think it's terrible the way some of these women talk about him. Why, I couldn't believe the things I heard. And the way he jokes and flirts with some of them..."

"He wants them to feel good."

"Well, he doesn't make me feel good. Lying here in bed all day long isn't good for me or for the baby, and the little ones at home need me."

"When Norma enters nurses' training at Good Samaritan, maybe you could have an X-ray taken there and get a second opinion." The room was beginning to darken and Mrs. Biddle who had the next bed, turned on her light.

"Doctor Sheridan won't let me go home for a visit. I guess he's afraid that I won't come back and I can't tell him that I want to see our family doctor. I'll think of something."

The door opened and Mrs. Kenny, the jolly, corpulent nurse who was working on the men's ward, came for Joe. "You're looking much better tonight," she commented, then nodded to Mrs. Darrell.

"Thanks, I feel much better even though my temperature is still a little high."

"You'll get to visit your mother again soon," she said, pushing the wheelchair toward the door.

"You're so busy. I do appreciate you coming for me, and getting away from the same four walls was relaxing. The visit with mother was wonderful."

He leaned against the back, watching the spokes of the wheel that whirred by his fingers and then the open doors. "There is an old girlfriend of mine here somewhere."

"What's her name?"

"Betty Gordon."

"I don't know her, but I'll try to find out where she is."

"Thank you. I would like to see her again sometime."

He heard the dull raps of her heels and the creaking of the old flooring as he rolled along and suddenly, he came to a stop by the nurses' desk and the drug room, just outside the sunporch. When he entered the sunporch, there were the horrifying memories of the past several months. The fellows who were playing poker talked in low voices: "Call, pass, up three..." They watched intently as pennies, nickels, and dimes slipped through their fingers and clinked against each other on the plastic top. In the second bed lay Randall, eyes closed, a rosary held in his hands. He was motionless except for the beads that slipped through his fingers. As he passed by the foot of the bed, Randall arose as if in a stupor, dragged his feet toward the windows, then leaned on the sill staring into an immensity of darkness, his mind going around and around with questions that were unanswerable. This phrenic that had paralyzed the left side of the diaphragm...how long would it last? And the heart pounding away with rapidity in its struggle to send life blood through the veins...the doctors, could they do nothing? What was it all about, this life? Only when he was a boy had there been any pleasure, any carefree, happy hours. These last ten years there had been no pleasure. He was waiting and waiting, but for what? The doctors? Come to me Lord...the Bible...the Bible...come to me Lord...

Slowly, he dragged himself to his bed and clasped the Bible. At last the stillness of the night moved in, but not for Randall. He sat up leaning forward, weaving and nodding, weaving and nodding, until his arms gave way and he lay flat on his face until the stiffness of his neck awakened him.

A shoving at his shoulder and a strange, raspy voice awakened Darrell. "Put this in your mouth and let me take your pulse."

He blinked and for a moment he thought his eyes were failing him.

Again she commanded, "Take this."

He looked up and standing there beside his bed was something that had walked out of a comic strip, or so he thought. Under droopy eyelids, one eye crossed through a pair of heavy, brown rimmed glasses. She had a long slender neck and wore a large man's watch on her bony wrist, and as she counted his pulse, he couldn't see whether she was looking at the watch or at him. Again he blinked his eyes.

She thought he was winking at her and a smile parted her bright red lips showing a slight gap between her uneven teeth.

"I could say something there," she said, staring down at him with one eye looking at Robbins. Finally, she turned and walked toward Skinner. She was working backward from the fifth bed toward the door.

"Isn't he cute, the little angel?" she said of Skinner who lay curled up like a ball, still asleep.

When she shoved a temp stick at him, he rubbed his eyes and began to yawn. Then he rubbed his eyes again. "Woe! A red-head! Wow!"

"I could say something there, but I won't," sounded her harsh notes.

The fellows looked from one to the other, roaring with laughter. Even Randall had joined in the laughter as she proceeded toward the door, her long spindly legs slapping her shoes against the floor in rapid succession as she swung her hips from side to side.

Darrell's eyes followed her through the door. "How would you like to wake up and find her in bed with you?" he asked.

"On a rainy night?" asked Bunnigan.

The fellows were still laughing and joking about her when Doctor Sheridan entered about an hour later.

"Sounds as if you fellows are having a grand time," he said, pausing at the foot of Randall's low bed.

Randall looked up sullenly. For more than a month the doctor had hurriedly passed him by with only a nod of his head or a few words.

"Your culture was negative," began the doctor, holding his chin. "Do you think some exercise might help you?"

Randall's face brightened momentarily. "I-I don't know! I'm very short of breath."

"It may help you to gain some strength," added the doctor. "I'll raise you to class two."

Then he paced to the dresser where he turned to glance about. Perhaps the laughter was good for them, he thought, and he was happy to report on the cultures performed on sputum samples taken more than six weeks ago.

"You were all negative on your last culture."

The faces of the fellows lit up while the doctor pondered,

"Bunnigan, do you think you're ready for class three?" Bunnigan smiled. Of course he was ready, and he handed his classification card to the doctor as he approached.

"I think I'm ready for class two," said Skinner.

The doctor chuckled. "You stay in that bed." And he laughed aloud, then nodded as he passed Darrell and quietly said, "You need more bed rest."

He raised Robbins to class three. The paraffin pack had helped. Leaving the room, he added with pride, "You fellows are all doing well."

"He must be sick," said Bunnigan.

"Must need more beds," remarked Darrell.

"But he didn't raise me in class," said Skinner.

Randall smiled. "We're all negative. Th-That hasn't happened to f-five in the same room since I've b-been here."

But things weren't to continue as rosy as they appeared to be. Randall welcomed the raise in class. His spirits were beaming with hope as he roamed through the halls visiting other patients, and he brought back the latest happenings and gossip. He joined in the laughter with the fellows who found the new nurse, Miss Klingland, to be cheerful and entertaining.

She flew about her work, her long spindly legs flapping loose-jointedly, and when she gave a bed bath, she handled the sheet carelessly and the washcloth more carelessly. Answering their remarks with: "I could say something there or, I could do something there." But she lacked the control over the fellows that Miss Sharen had. Consequently, there was more buffoonery and more poker sessions started by Transfusion and Bunnigan in the evenings.

In one of his rare moods, Transfusion entered waving his arms. "Come on you loafers! Take the cash in hand. We are here but to play and die, so unless one of you witty bums has a better solution, let's go!" He continued to wave his arms like a Shakespearean character. "You know the road. It's this-a-way. Come on you bums!"

"Ahoy there mates," shouted Bunnigan, climbing out of bed, always ready for a poker game. "To the crow's nest, you buzzards! Gib the sails. Man the sheets! You heard what the little admiral said."

Skinner raised his thumb to his nose as he stood up in bed.

'"Aye, Aye, Captain," he sang, then peering out across the porch to the leeward side with a hand to his forehead and the other pointing, he shouted, "Thar she blows!"

Then Transfusion waved his arms wildly, and began to sing:

"Yo ho, blow the man down bullies,
Blow the man down...
Yo ho, give him some time
to blow the man down..."

Darrell was lucky in cards and he enjoyed playing poker, but his temperature remained over 100 and the heavy perspiration continued. It was with a real sense of concern for his health and in keeping with the doctor's request that he remained in bed. He hoped that the high temperature and the heavy perspiration would help him to recover. With the recent drop in his fever, he felt much better.

Their clowning was cut short when Miss Sharen returned from her two-week vacation, however the fellows welcomed her. She proudly displayed the engagement ring, which she had received from Doctor Harman. She was full of excitement with the thoughts and plans of her forthcoming wedding, which was to take place in October. She continued to perform her work with the same dedicated diligence and cheerfulness. The fellows had become more acquainted with, and accustomed to, Miss Klingland. She was a good-natured nurse and her assistance on the surgery ward was welcomed. The fellows would have preferred to have Miss Downley. She had left the sanatorium and none of the patients had heard anything about her whereabouts.

Darrell had visited his mother again and she had planned a visit home for the first of September. She had obtained that permission with the promise of returning in three days. She had none of the symptoms of any infection and the women couldn't understand what she was doing here. In her situation it was a means of segregation to free the children from infection that had no merit.

There was no need for careful observation. State and county health departments were limited in their activities and inadequately trained and staffed, and in Mrs. Darrell's situation it was made to appear absolutely necessary for complete segregation and careful observation which imposed a real hardship on the family. It gave to the health department a sense of importance and it portrayed it as a protector in the eyes of the community that appeared to be beyond question in the case of Mrs. Darrell. It created a cause of deep concern and worry for Mr. Darrell, and for Joe it created a needless feeling of guilt and deep responsibility. So it was with some relief when his mother told him that she would see their family doctor when she was home.

Occasionally, a minister from one of the local churches would visit the patients in the sanatorium and this time Darrell was awakened from the afternoon rest hour promptly at three o'clock by the high soprano voices that drifted through the second floor men's ward. For a moment he didn't realize where he was as the words rang out: "...I'll be safe in the arms of Jesus..."

He looked about. Bunnigan was lying there with his eyes closed and Randall was staring at the ceiling in meditation. Skinner began to sing along and then he suddenly blurted, "For I am Jesus' little lamb! Yes, by Jesus Christ I am!"

A minister began to preach as Miss Sharen, wearing a solemn expression, entered the room to take the afternoon pulses and temperatures.

"...The Lord is your Shepherd; He helpeth you to lie down and rest. He will make your days and nights bright with his presence. Lift up your mind and heart to him so that you may be healed..."

The nurse was taking Skinner's pulse. "That's what I'll do," mumbled Skinner.

"Why, Skinner?" said Miss Sharen, trying to keep a serious face.

"...The light of ever-present love is all-powerful," continued the minister. "We mortals are but the reflection of the infinite Being..."

Skinner raised his voice. "That's what I told them."

Randall glared at Skinner. "Not so loud."

"...Each or us reflects the spiritual qualities in his mind. God is the mind. Lift your heart to the mind...not my will but thine be done...let us pray...Our Father which art in heaven..."

After the Lord's Prayer, Rev. Ragen, from one of the local churches, visited the fellows on the sunporch carrying under one arm a collection of periodicals. When he offered Randall a copy, he shook his head, for Randall didn't think or believe it was right for him to read any other literature pertaining to religion than that of his own faith. His smile and the nod of his head shielded the blank expression that crossed the minister's ruddy face as he turned toward Bunnigan who had the bed in the corner by the windows.

Bunnigan thanked the minister for the literature. "When I think about the mind and religion, I go around in circles. There are so many different religions and churches, each with their own righteous teachings and beliefs and ways to get to heaven, that I wind up where I started—without religion."

The minister gave Bunnigan a questioning glance. "Your mind governs your spiritual well-being as well as your physical well-being. The choice is yours. We must have a strong desire, the God-given mental power, a will for survival if you wish."

"That's what my wife said," commented Bunnigan, "until she read about the theory of evolution and the survival of the fittest. We're not the fittest, but weaklings."

"Evidently, your wife doesn't understand," said the minister, who had started toward Skinner.

Skinner accepted a tabloid out of curiosity.

"My wife understands," said Bunnigan in a derisive tone.

Rev. Ragen had started to walk toward Robbins. He paused for a moment. "Bless her," he said. As he walked there seemed to be a domineering note about his carriage, and yet his manners were complaisant. His white starched collar was outstanding atop his oxford gray suit. Bobbins accepted the literature out of courtesy. He had no intentions of reading any of it.

Your sermon was most heartening," said Darrell, accepting a copy of the small tabloid.

Darrell came from a religious family. Throughout his school years, eight in grade school and four years in high school, his parents made that extra effort, expense, and sacrifice to see that the children arrived at school in time to attend morning mass prior to school. And in the winter time when he was in the lower grades, it was still dark on many a cold morning when his father left Joe and his sister Mary at the school on his way to work. He had heard many a sermon, but none quite like this one about the mind and physical well-being.

"Thank you. It was meant to set your mind at ease," said the minister as he stepped back taking a sideward glance through his rimless glasses toward Randall and Bunnigan.

Before leaving the room, the minister paused at the side of Bunnigan's bed. "We'll continue our discussion at a later date."

Randall watched indifferently as the minister spoke a few words with the elderly maid who was waiting to enter the room to begin her cleaning.

As soon as the minister had stepped out of the room, Skinner crumpled the periodical that he had received and threw it toward the wastebasket that stood near the dresser. "Sounds like double talk to me; all this stuff about the mind. Does he think that's all there is wrong with us?"

The elderly maid who was about to turn on the vacuum cleaner, waved the attached hose around her head and pointed the metal-flared brush at Skinner. "How can you say that? Haven't you read the Bible?"

"Yeah, I read the Old Testament once, but that New Testament, you can't believe that."

Randall sat up in bed and began to sputter. ""Bu-bu-bu-but-but, that isn't true. You ca-can trace it from history."

"A pack of lies," grumbled Skinner as the fellows roared with laughter.

When the maid heard this she started the sweeper in a roaring huff, and turned it off again as Randall began to stammer.

"'Bu-bu-but, I wouldn't say that about your Bible, or wh-wh-whatever the Rabbi gave you when, when he was here. Rabbi Neuheim, he-he carries that cane and wears that goatee to-to look like a-a, Solomon."

"I don't say anything about the priest who comes every

Sunday morning and gives you and Darrell that little cracker or whatever you call it," taunted Skinner.

Randall's face was very red and he was gasping for breath. He started to stammer again when Darrell tried to calm the atmosphere. "What's the argument about?"

It was Bunnigan's delight to keep the argument going. "The different Bibles that contradict themselves."

"To each his own," said Darrell.

The elderly maid, who the fellows called "California", jumped astraddle the hose and turned toward Bunnigan with the hose pulling against her leg and skirt as she waved the metal attachment.

"Now, that isn't so at all. There is only one Bible and everything that the Bible mentions has happened. You know it has," she said, untangling the hose from her leg.

"More superstition," grumbled Skinner.

"Do you believe there is a heaven?" taunted Bunnigan.

"Well, sure there is. The Bible says so. My brother in California is a minister and he showed..."

"Ho, ho, ho-o..." bellowed Bunnigan, an agnostic who believed only what he thought he could or what suited the circumstance.

"He showed me in the Bible that there is," added the maid.

"I wish that my belief was as strong as yours. I'd be ready to die anytime. Ho, ho, ho-o."

Randall had a worried look upon his face and held one hand over his heart.

Skinner interrupted Bunnigan. "You heard what the Rev. said. 'Raise up your mind and you will get well.'"

"Yes, it's so simple," said Darrell. "If we would only do that, then we wouldn't be here and there wouldn't be any need for hospitals."

The elderly maid shook her head hopelessly as she continued her cleaning.

"I wish I knew what to believe," continued Bunnigan in a more serious tone. "Because when my daughter grows up I would like to see her go to church, but there are so many that I don't know which one."

"Here's your opportunity to find out," said Robbins. "Most every month a minister of some church visits the patients and sometimes more often."

"I haven't heard any singing or sermons before today," said Darrell. Is this something new?"

"The singing was an added feature," remarked Robbins, "and we usually hear a sermon once a month. This was the week for the second floor men's ward."

"That's too often for me," said Skinner.

Late that evening, after the shadows of night had crept in upon the porch, Randall took out his rosary and prayed with all his heart and soul. And at night a thousand thoughts came to him as he sat up in bed struggling for breath. The continual struggle was a drain upon his energy and he sank deeper with his despondency, but every afternoon he read his Bible ardently. As the doctor made his rounds, he passed him by swiftly. The fellows shook their heads and asked each other why something couldn't be done for him. Doctor Sheridan had tried all that medical science had to offer. Randall was negative, but he had difficulty obtaining his breath; his phrenic was doing its work. The lungs had to be kept at rest. Diet and bed rest alone were not sufficient. The bacilli were lodged in old lesions established over a period of years. Chemotherapy didn't exist. Randall did his best to regain some strength as Doctor Sheridan had suggested. His exercise, consistent with the raise to class two, consisted mainly of the daily trips to and from the bathroom and he would return to his bed panting for breath.

The recent raise to class three meant more activity for Bunnigan than bathroom privileges. Many times in the late evening hours when Eve Stevens was on duty, he would steal away with a book in hand for a rendezvous with her. She was well read, he said, and he enjoyed talking with her about the books they read, the activities at the sanatorium, and their secret romance.

About this time, after almost two months of high temperature, Darrell's temperature dropped to normal. What a wonderful feeling it was. Gradually he was able to eat more of the solid foods. His diaphragm had risen on his right side and his lung was forcing its way out. He received pneumos after his side was aspirated and irrigated with the Azocloramid solution, to hold as much air space as possible and to prevent the lung from sticking to his pleural wall. It also helped to control the empyema and kept the upper lobe of his lung at rest.

After further inquiry about Betty Gordon, Darrell had learned from Mrs. Kenny, the night nurse, that she had a relapse. She had been in class ten or eleven. It was the second time around. She was in the second floor sunroom, which was located on the far east wing. Through Mrs. Kenny he managed to visit her. She was in good spirits, but couldn't understand why she had a positive culture. She talked about the long walks around the lake which was only a short distance away, and she believed that the exercise was too much and too soon. "But such is life in the sanatorium," she said. The visit was brief and pleasant under the circumstances, as Mrs. Kenny talked with some of the other patients in the sunroom.

Chapter XIII

DARRELL'S MOTHER RECEIVES A SECOND OPINION

In the red, brick farm house near Celina, an active mother was busily engaged checking the children's wardrobe for the school year that was about to commence. Norma listened attentively as she gave the last minute instructions, however no one could replace the maternal care.

"Is Daddy ready to go?" asked Mother.

"Daddy is waiting in the car," replied Norma.

"Keep the little ones in the kitchen, Norma," she whispered, "so they won't see me leaving."

The kitchen door opened; little five year old Barbi stood there staring.

"I want to go with you, Mother."

"Hurry, take them into the kitchen before it's too late."

"I want to go," said Barbi, pleadingly.

"I'll be back, Barbi. Do as Norma says," she commanded as she hurried out the door.

"Don't cry," said Bernadette. "Mother is going to the hospital."

Before she had finished, Barbi was crying. Then the two smaller children joined in with loud crying and wailing.

Upon her return to the sanatorium, Mrs. Darrell, accompanied by her husband, stopped on the sunporch to visit their son. Under her light fall coat, her pregnancy was less pronounced.

"You appear rested after your visit home," remarked Joe as they approached.

"And you have more color than you did," commented Mr. Darrell.

"I've gained five pounds in the past month and my fluid is almost gone."

"Does it affect everyone that way?" asked Mrs. Darrell.

"The majority, but there are exceptions. Some patients eat more and even feel better. Sometimes the fluid actually helps. It's nature's way of combating TB, but I don't know what it did for me." After the pause that followed, Joe asked, "How was everything at home?"

"When I got home the little ones came running out of the house yelling, 'Mother is home! Mother is home! Home to stay! Home to stay!' I could hardly get to the house. They were pulling and tugging at my dress. And Nita who is just starting to walk, didn't even know or recognize me. She began to cry, and she is so puny and thin."

"What did Doctor Hattery say?"

"He said, 'Why, you don't have any more TB than that chair.'"

Mrs. Darrell laughed, then continued, "He told me that a woman's lungs sometimes appear a little cloudy when she is carrying a child."

"Did you talk to Doctor Sheridan yet?"

"He disagrees—says that in my case, there were some changes from one X-ray to the next."

"He won't even listen," added Mr. Darrell, disgustedly. "I tried to tell him that it was because of the added rest."

"Did you talk to the health department?"

"Doctor Hattery will," said Mr. Darrell.

"Daddy didn't want me to come back at all, but I had promised."

"You aren't staying though, are you?"

"I'll have to have another talk with Doctor Sheridan. Norma wants to leave for nurses' training and then I should be home, because there will be no one to take care of the little ones."

As they were leaving for the sunroom on the first floor, she added, "I'll let you know what the future will bring."

Although the days continued rather hot, the nights and especially the early mornings, were cool and crisp. It was good sleeping weather after a long hot summer of sweaty nights. A sudden coolness and a heavy frost followed an early autumn rain. The days were becoming shorter and the leaves of the various trees were changing to a brilliant hue, making a colorful landscape beneath the clear autumn skies.

By mid-September, Bunnigan and Robbins, who had been in class four for three weeks, were raised to class five and transferred to the new building. That afternoon, Doctor Sheridan paid an unexpected visit to Randall.

"Do you think that oxygen would help you to rest better?" he asked in a discerning voice.

Randall wasn't quick to reply. His thoughts were of those that he knew who had previously been forced to use oxygen—rarely did they recover.

"You have had your phrenic now for seven months," continued the doctor. "Until your diaphragm becomes active again, the oxygen will help you to breath and rest better."

Randall looked up through bloodshot and tired eyes, and there was only a faint smile. "All right," he said very quietly. He was forced to sit up in bed more frequently and longer now. There was no choice.

"I'll have a tank sent up," he said, turning slowly away.

Fifteen minutes later, a porter wheeled a large green, steel tank onto the porch. No sooner had he set the tank off his two-wheeled cart, Miss Sharen entered.

"Mr. Randall, isn't the doctor going to move you to a private room?"

Randall didn't like the thought of leaving the porch for a private room. He enjoyed the company of Darrell and Skinner in spite of all their jokes. He was deeply saddened and it showed on his face. He answered with a shrug of his shoulders.

"There is one vacant," she said, frowning as she looked from Darrell, who was now in the first bed, to Skinner. "These fellows wouldn't be allowed to smoke while you're using oxygen."

Randall did not reply. He was deeply hurt. He would miss their companionship.

Darrell looked at Randall with compassion. "Maybe we could quit smoking. It would be better for us. I'd try."

"Me too," said Skinner.

The nurse knew better. "Gene, wouldn't you rather be in a private room?"

"I guess so," he answered as he looked from Darrell to Skinner.

"Wait here," she said to the porter as she left the room. Until yesterday, Mr. Fornay who had hemorrhaged and died had occupied the private room.

The porter, a short restless fellow, mumbled, "These nurses always wanting to change things when they don't have to do the work. Just like my wife always moving the furniture around."

Miss Sharen returned saying, "The doctor meant to have you moved."

The porter already had the container on his cart and headed for the vacant room. From the bed in the corner, Darrell could see through the glass doors of the sunporch across the corridor to the vacant private room where Randall was being moved.

California, the elderly maid, was helping him move his meager belongings and Skinner's bed was moved into the place that Randall had occupied. After the exchange of beds, the porch seemed quiet and strange. Only Skinner and Darrell remained. Doctor Sheridan entered the room as Miss Sharen was adjusting the gauge and taping the tube to Randall's upper lip.

"Only use it when you feel that you need it," said the doctor.

That evening Transfusion was forced to venture downstairs to find a few poker players. He returned in a short while. "You'd think they were all dying downstairs. Can't even get a game started. Doc sure ruined our poker games when he transferred Bunnigan and Robbins."

"Yes, I believe he knew that we had some good poker sessions going," commented Darrell. "Let's go over and see how Randall is doing."

"Say, did you guys hear about Towers?" asked Transfusion.

"No," replied Darrell and Skinner in unison as they were climbing out of their beds.

"When I was downstairs, I heard that Towers had a positive sputum check. I guess that put the fear into them. They were a gloomy looking bunch of doom sayers."

There was a sudden, deep compassionate feeling of sympathy and grief that encompassed them as they stared from one to the other. Towers had received the best medical attention that was available at that time, and the best food and diet.

"I think he had a real fear of the exercise that he was required to take as he progressed in the classes," said Darrell. "As a consequence, the exercise became more worrisome and detrimental for him."

"He was in class ten," said Skinner, shaking his head as they proceeded toward the first private room on the right.

Randall was resting comfortably with his head propped against two pillows. He looked up from his Bible and gave a huge smile as the fellows entered the room. The tube was taped above his upper lip and extended up one nostril.

"He's got some color in his cheeks," commented Transfusion. There was a happy smile and a gleam in Randall's eyes. "This is what I needed."

"How much are you supposed to use?" queried Darrell.

"As much as I need," replied Randall. "I use it for fifteen minutes and then turn it off for fifteen. I feel a world of difference."

"He's coming up in the world," bantered Skinner.

"Yes, he's back in a high bed again," said Darrell.

That night Skinner and Darrell listened to their radios until after the ten o'clock news broadcast. The three empty beds added to the ghastly shadows as ominous coughs re-echoed through the darkness. From above the door to the first cubbyhole, a light gleamed throughout the transom. There, Mrs. Kenny gave Transfusion a hypo as she did every two hours through the night. Skinner's voice echoed in the stillness. "It's strange on the porch without Randall."

"I keep looking over there expecting to see Randall sitting up in bed," added Darrell. "Of the original five, we are now down to two. I wonder how Bunnigan and Robbins are doing, and how they like the new building?"

Skinner had spent more than a year at the new building. "It's a nice place. There's no comparison with this surgery ward."

Darrell rolled over on his right side. "Randall looked better tonight than he has for a long time."

"Yeah, better than he has for nine months since we've shared this same porch."

"He didn't stammer tonight, did you notice?"

"He needed oxygen bad," said Skinner.

"I wonder why Doc didn't give it to him sooner. He was getting worse day by day."

"There were no private rooms available."

"And I suppose Doc felt the exercise would help him, and that he would make it without oxygen," said Darrell sleepily, and added, "Wonder who'll be moved into the other beds?"

"Probably Towers, for one."

"From class ten to class one and a half? That's really tough to take and this is his third time around."

"With this stuff, a guy never knows."

"Towers worries too much, though he doesn't show it," added Darrell.

Their voices dragged somnolently and sleep soon overtook them.

Hours passed. Then through the still night, a booming voice re-echoed through the corridors. Darrell and Skinner sat upright and listened closely to the reverberating voice.

"...The Lord is my shepherd; I shall not want. He maketh me to lie down in green pastures: he leadeth me beside the still waters. He restoreth my soul. He leadeth me in the paths of righteousness for his namesake. Yea, though I walk through the valley of the shadow of death, I will fear no evil, for thou art with me..."

"That sounds like the preacher giving a sermon," said Skinner as he pulled the covers around his shoulders."

The loud voice grew in intensity. Darrell shivered and looked about as he reached for his blankets. It was very dark outside. He looked through the glass doors at the lighted corridor. The voice sounded a little like Randall's voice, but very strong and loud.

"...Forsake me not, O Lord. O my God, be not far from me..." continued the loud voice, growing louder and louder.

"There's a light in Randall's room," said Darrell.

"Must be reading the Bible," added Skinner.

"He doesn't stammer. His voice is so strong. It's much stronger and louder than the preacher's voice."

Heavy, hurried footsteps were rapidly approaching as the reverberating voice continued loud and clear.

"Doctor Sheridan just rounded the corridor," said Darrell. As the door opened and the doctor entered, Darrell saw Randall wildly waving his arms, the Bible in one hand and his eyes glaring through his brown rimmed glasses with a hideous stare as his voice echoed even louder.

"Come to me Lord. Come to me Lord."

The door closed and opened again as Mrs. Kenny, the night nurse, hurried to the drug room and returned closing the door behind her.

A loud slap reverberated, then another and another. Randall's voice boomed, strong and firm: "Stand back. Stand back."

Then another slap followed by another.

"Don't touch me. Don't touch me," echoed Randall, clear and loud without any hesitation and his voice boomed forth again, piercing the stilled night. "Come to me Lord. Come to me Lord."

Again the slapping and again the booming voice.

Darrell and Skinner looked from one to the other. Then they lay down and waited, covering their heads. The strong booming voice rang in their ears and grew fainter and fainter. A cold chill ran over them. Their teeth chattered and their nerves trembled and quivered until they tired of exhaustion. Finally sleep moved in once more.

Chapter XIV

TWO NEW PATIENTS

The dawn that broke was cool and crisp. Later than usual, Miss Sharen appeared on the sunporch, silent and glum. As she was taking Darrell's pulse, he glanced toward the door. A stretcher rumbled through the corridor with the body that she had prepared for the morgue, pushed by the little porter who had wheeled the green cylinder tank of oxygen into the room yesterday. She shook her head as tears filled her eyes. Randall's voice clear and loud, rang in his ears—his calls for help and life. It had all ended so suddenly. The routine of the day followed as usual. When Doctor Sheridan appeared that morning, his head hung with sorrow. He had done all that he possibly could and his voice was mournful. Darrell obtained permission to visit his mother and after the doctor had left, he tried to read, but the book trembled in his hands. He was shaken by the experience.

When he arrived at his mother's room, it was after seven that evening. The women had already heard about Randall, but they wanted more detail and he related his experience of the previous night. It helped to relieve the tension that had gripped his nerves.

A discussion followed and one thing led to another.

"One of the nurses broke down," said Mrs. Tice, the thin woman in the corner. "I was at the office today and couldn't help but overhear her talking to Sheridan. He wants her to enter the sanatorium for rest and maybe pneumothorax treatment if her X-ray doesn't clear."

He was thinking about his mother's X-ray. "Which nurse was it?"

"You all know her," continued Mrs. Tice. "She worked on this ward part of the time and she was always so neat and pleasant...a Miss Downley. She was heartbroken when Doctor Harman left."

"Miss Downley!" said Joe, interrupting, and a pause followed.

"She was the nurse who told me that you were feeling sick from your fluid," remarked his mother, "but that I needn't worry; you would be all right."

He sat there as if he were in a stupor. Mary Jane Downley!

"That was the last time I saw her."

"It's been about two months," continued Mrs. Tice, "and she's been trying to rest at home. Sheridan said that he wanted her to have the best of care and that as soon as he has a private room available, she would have it."

Hundreds of thoughts ran through his mind as the women continued to talk.

"Doctor Sheridan doesn't want me to leave," said his mother, breaking into his thoughts. "He keeps joking about the baby. Says he hasn't delivered any for quite some time. Why, I wouldn't have him on a bet. The very thought of having a baby born here. Wait until Daddy gets here Sunday."

Mrs. Kenny entered and as he was wheeled back to the sunporch, they talked about Miss Downley. She said that Miss Downley wasn't really as sick as the women believed. He felt somewhat better and hoped that he might see her again, for she had been so very kind to him.

The following day about eleven in the morning, Towers returned to the sunporch. Bunnigan and Robbins came along to visit with Skinner and Darrell and to learn more about what had happened to Randall. After Darrell and Skinner had related as much as they could of their gruesome experience, Bunnigan asked, "Which of Doc's prize patients will be next?"

Towers, who was feeling in very low spirits, replied, "That isn't funny, Bub."

No further comments were made about Randall and in an attempt to relieve some of the tension, Darrell, remembering the day that he had entered, asked, "How long did Doc say you'd have to be in?"

Towers, seated on the edge of the third bed, gave a surprised look and then laughed. "About eight months."

"Well, I see you haven't forgotten."

When the laughter faded, Robbins said, "You ought to be due for a raise in class."

Darrell shook his head. "Not until I have another X-ray, and that's not for six weeks."

"How about you Skinner?"

"I should be. I'm going to ask Doc one of these days."

"You keep asking him," bantered Bunnigan, "and he'll get tired of telling you to stay in that bed."

"How's your fluid, Darrell?" asked Towers.

"It's gone, but I can only take 100 cc's of air."

Mary Boswell entered carrying a small zipper bag. A tall, dark-haired fellow, who looked to be in his late thirties or early forties, followed her. Deep wrinkles lined his cheeks and his brow as he frowned while he listened to the superintendent of nurses who was speaking quietly. After she showed him his locker, he took out a pair of pajamas and followed her toward the bathroom.

"Well," said Towers as he climbed into bed, "at least, we'll have somebody new. We'll give him the works."

There was a clattering of dishes in the corridor. "Say, we've got to get going or we'll miss our dinner," remarked Robbins to Bunnigan.

"See you guys," said Bunnigan, and added, "Don't be too rough on the new victim."

"Yeah, we'll be around here for awhile," called Skinner as they were leaving.

The tall, dark-haired fellow returned wearing a wine-colored robe that stopped short of his knees. He looked sternly about him, then draped the robe over a chair by the fourth bed and climbed between the sheets that the nurse had turned back. There was a gaunt look about him, evident of the loss of weight. "Mr. Marrow," called Miss Sharen, entering the room, "what would you like to drink, milk, coffee, or tea?"

"Coffee," he replied in a low tone.

"Wouldn't you like a glass of milk too?"

"Yes, maam," he replied after some thought.

"Where 'ya from?" queried Towers, who had the bed next to Marrow.

"South of Bellfountain."

Towers nodded his head. "What's new in Bellfountain?"

"With the war on, the factories are going full blast. It's a lively place."

"Here you are, Mr. Marrow," said Miss Sharen. "Do you want your bed raised?"

"Yes, maam." The nurse set the tray at the foot of his bed while she raised the head and then placed the tray over the small bed table.

The questions were discontinued until after dinner and while Marrow waited for his bed to be lowered, he asked, "How do you guys manage to sit up and eat that way?"

Towers gave a chuckle. "After you've been here awhile, it's relaxing to get your back off the bed."

"How long have you been in?"

"Just a little over two years."

"What? Two years!" he gasped and his mouth dropped open.

"That's nothing," said Skinner. "This is my second cure. I've been here four years."

Marrow shook his head distressfully.

"Darrell, the fellow in the corner bed," said Towers, "hasn't been here very long."

"Seven months!" injected Darrell. "Doc said that I might be out in eight months. It sounds like a prison sentence."

Marrow frowned and the fellows laughed.

"How did you find out about it?" asked Darrell.

"During my army physical, but I knew that I wasn't feeling well. I was working two jobs and I couldn't eat right. My stomach was upset and I felt nervous. When I went to the doctor, he gave me some pills to quiet my nerves and settle my stomach. He told me to quit one of my jobs and get some more sleep. At that time I was working in a dairy."

"In a dairy!" interrupted Skinner, "those bugs ought to grow well."

"Well, at least the cows are required to be inspected in order to eliminate infection from bovine sources," said Darrell. "Our cows on the farm have metal tags clipped in their ears to certify that they were inspected."

"What did you do on the other job?" asked Towers.

"Worked in a butcher shop."

Towers chuckled. "My, oh my, how the bugs will travel. You couldn't have worked in better spots."

Marrow sighed. "I had to work. I've got a family to support."

"We all worked," began Towers. "I graduated from Ohio State and had a good position with an accounting firm there. One of the fellows who worked with me broke down. I thought, hell it won't happen to me and I didn't think much about it. If I had enough sense to have an X-ray taken sooner, I wouldn't be here now."

Darrell was thinking the same about himself. "At Patterson Field some of us had to work alternate shifts. I never could sleep properly and on the night owl shift about four in the morning, I could hardly stay awake. If the doctor had properly diagnosed this phthisis, as some doctors call it, I wouldn't be here either."

"Call it what they want," continued Towers. "This is my second time in. The first year that I was at Mount Vernon. The folks would come to see me occasionally, but now, after almost four years, I'm lucky if I see them once a year. My uncle comes almost every other month. He and I are still good friends."

Marrow wiped his brow. "Four years!"

"Rest hour," called Miss Sharen from the doorway.

The afternoon rest hour ended their talk and Marrow sank deeper and deeper with a thousand gloomy thoughts.

When Transfusion rushed onto the porch late that afternoon, Marrow's dark eyes looked as if they were ready to pop.

"Did you guys see the black wagon?" he asked as his steps slowed.

The fellows climbed out of their beds and gathered along the windows. Even Marrow who was supposed to have complete rest was there, peering down at the black hearse that crept to a stop below.

"Who are they after?" he asked.

"The fellow who had your bed until two nights ago," sounded Skinner's.

"He was a nice guy too," added Darrell. "He read his Bible every day most ardently."

Marrow's black heavy brows were drawn together in a frown.

"There he is!" said Towers.

"The sure cure!" added Transfusion, "Toes up!"

"After ten years of struggling," added Darrell, "the operation was a success, but the patient died."

"Ten years!" gasped Marrow.

"Yep, and then some," replied Transfusion with a chuckle and followed it by a hacking cough.

Marrow watched as he took out the folded cup and cleared his throat, and then after careful scrutiny, Transfusion folded the cup and put it in his pocket. With his other hand he brushed the hair out of his eyes, then chuckled, "Ah-a, that was a good one!"

"What are they doing for you?" asked Marrow.

"Not a damn thing, but give me a hypo every two hours to keep my cough down. I'm just hanging around. I had a cure once, if you could call it that, and when I was out I made up my mind that if I ever broke down again, I would go as long and as far as I could." His Adam's apple bobbed up and down while he chuckled, "Well I did, and they carried me in here on a stretcher after I was shipped from California." Again he chuckled, "California didn't want me. I ruined their environment."

It seemed incredible that he had such an attitude and that such an attitude could exist. This was certainly no way to control the disease. It was dangerous to the community and the health of everyone with whom he came in contact. The public didn't know how to protect themselves. Laws were inadequate to protect the public and as a consequence, society was saturated with active carriers. These unfortunates were those who had been subjected to unhealthy circumstances. Many of the states had not provided hospital care. Sanatorium space and beds were very limited. There was always the problem of financial aid. Funds from the sale of Christmas seals had provided much help in educational work, the organization and operation of clinics, and in the establishment of TB divisions in the health departments. However, little had been accomplished in a preventive way. TB societies had struggled on in the hope that physicians would find TB infection early through diagnostic methods. These were inadequate and there were differences in medical opinions, as was now apparent in Mrs. Darrell's situation.

"You were fortunate that Ohio took you back," said Marrow shaking his head and climbing back into bed. The following day Marrow received his first pneumo. It wasn't as successful as it should have been. There wasn't much pressure and he didn't feel any ill effects. After two days of rest he appeared to feel somewhat better, however his mood was worse, very gloomy. When Sunday came, his wife visited him. She wore a plain cotton dress, and there was a sincere and concerned look about her as she talked with him about their five children and how she was going to make ends meet. She planned to obtain work in one of the local factories and the youngest child would have to go to nursery school. The children's ages ranged from four to fourteen. The stories he had heard, and what little that he knew about tuberculosis, made him feel very depressed. She didn't stay very long, for she began to weep and left the room in tears.

That Sunday, Mr. Darrell stopped to visit.

"I'm taking Mother home today," he said. "Mother said that she had a nice visit with you and she won't be able to see you before she leaves."

"Did you talk to Doctor Sheridan?"

Mr. Darrell's eyes flashed with disapproval and sorrow, and Joe was sorry that he could do nothing, since he felt that he was to blame for all the trouble and problems caused by his mother being here.

"I've talked with him before and Mother has talked with him. He doesn't agree and his opinion is just opposed to Doctor Hattery. I talked to Hattery again. He said that Mother should have never been here. He can't understand it and neither can I. It will be much better for Mother to be home, Doctor Hattery said.

Mother has never coughed or had any of the symptoms. The children need Mother."

Mr. Darrell arose and walked to the windows at the foot of Joe's bed. "I have the car parked around near her room. You can see the rear of the car from here. It's close to the nurses' building.

Your car is running better than ours."

Joe peered from the windows that ran alongside his bed. Four little tots were jumping around on the rear seat of his old gray '38 Chevy.

"Mother ought to be ready. Maybe you'll be able to get home soon."

"I'll soon be feeling stronger than I do now. I was weaker than a kitten."

"Mother will be much better at home," Mr. Darrell said as he was leaving the room, then paused saying, "and Norma left last week for nurses' training at Good Samaritan Hospital in Dayton."

That evening he wrote a letter to Pat. He explained some of the happenings—the death of Randall, his mother's departure, and his progress and concern for her, since he hadn't heard from her in several weeks.

When Doctor Sheridan entered the room the following morning, he expected him to comment on his mother's leaving without permission.

"How do you feel, Mr. Marrow?" he asked.

"All right," nodded Marrow, as if nothing was wrong.

"We'll fluoroscope you tomorrow and see if we can give you another pneumo. We didn't get much air in on your first pneumo." He paused and Marrow nodded again. Then the doctor continued with a laugh, "Don't listen to everything that these guys tell you." He glanced about from Towers, to Skinner, and to Darrell before he added, "I have a young fellow coming in this afternoon for that corner bed and I want you fellows to lay off.

We don't have any private rooms available and we don't want him frightened to death."

Doctor Sheridan was no more than out of the room when Skinner began with a laugh, "That's just what we need—somebody to pour it on."

"Marrow, you'll see how it's done," said Towers.

"We were easy on you," added Darrell, "just like Doc requested."

He entered that afternoon, a young fellow, about twenty-two. He was apparently another army reject. He had light brown hair and eyes, and a lanky frame that needed filling. His eyes opened wide as the old lungers began to pour it on as soon as he told them that Doc had said that he would be out in six months. The same routine followed—four years for Towers, four years for Skinner, and seven months for Darrell, and they continued in serious tones.

"Do you have a cavity?" asked Towers.

The new unfortunate victim, Mr. Blande, nodded. "I have two," he said as if he were proud of the fact, or as if it were something to brag about. "One is the size of a quarter and the other is about the size of a nickel or a little larger."

"Oh, my hell!" exclaimed Skinner, patting his curly hair, "Two cavities!"

"I had one smaller than a dime that Doc could hardly see," bantered Towers, "and I've been in here for four years. Let's see, for you that figures out to be eight years!"

"And he thought he would be out in six months," added Skinner with a laugh.

"Yo, ho, ho-o...." And all three joined in the laughter.

Marrow stared at the three old lungers with a serious face, as did Blande, while they roared all the louder.

"Doc will give you pneumos for them," jeered Darrell.

"There's really nothing to 'em."

"What are they?"

"Well let's see. Doc had better tell you about them," answered Darrell.

Blande persisted. "What are they?"

Towers looked serious for the moment. "Doc's got a long needle, about as long as my index, or maybe a little l-o-n-g-e-r," he replied, holding up a long slender finger, "and Doc's got you strapped to the stretcher as tight as they can pull the straps, so you can't get away. He jabs that long needle right up your rib.

Then he pumps you full of air."

Skinner opened the top of his pajamas. Fresh needle marks and scars were visible. "I was fourteen when I got my first pneumo. My uncle came to the clinic to watch and when Doc jabbed me with the needle, my uncle passed out. Yo, ho, ho-o..."

Blande stared at them with a half-grin as the fellows roared.

"Sometimes they get so much air that it pushes the shoulder three inches higher than the other one and it never comes down," remarked Darrell, then added, "Remember the fellow who passed away...I mean, died when Doc hit a nerve? The pneumothorax was successful, but he couldn't breathe or his heart stopped."

Towers was shaking his head with sorrow. "He was a young fellow too. And not only that," continued Towers in a serious tone, "if pneumos aren't successful, Doc's going to make you a Christmas present, all clean and pickled in alcohol, nine of your own ribs."

The day that Blande received his first pneumo, he lay there with anger in his eyes and groaned and coughed, opening his mouth wide with loud whooping bellows. It wasn't good for his lungs. Marrow turned his stern eyes upon him and for spite, he bellowed all the more, even though Marrow had said nothing when the fellows were pouring it on.

Blande was in class one the same as Marrow, and every

morning the curtains were pulled while they sat upon the thrones, as Towers had called the commodes. Though the windows were open, the perfume was enough to drive the three old lungers away from "Commodilly Row". Darrell made a sign and hung it on one of the curtains: "Danger Ahead-Men Blastin'!"

With the arrival of the new patients, Darrell overcame the nervous tension that Randall had caused. His thoughts drifted freely and his attitude was good. He looked forward to the time when he would be able to take some exercise. He was occupied more than before with thoughts of concern for Pat since he had not heard from her recently. He also had thoughts of Miss Downley, until that day toward the last of September when the preacher's voice boomed loudly through the corridors.

"...The Lord is your Shepherd; He..."

"That sounds like Randall! It is strange how similar. It gives me gooseflesh," said Darrell as he slipped out of bed and into his robe.

"Yeah, that voice gives me the creeps," said Skinner. "Let's get the hell out of here."

They left through the door of the last cubbyhole as if they were being chased while Towers, Marrow, and Blande watched in astonishment and alarm. The words drifted through the corridor. They entered the large antechamber at the bathroom, but the door could not be closed and the sound echoed.

"It does sound like Randall's voice," said Skinner, "and almost the same words too."

"What a strange coincidence," said Darrell. "The same words and phrasing and that sound; it really gives me the jitters. After seven months of sharing the same room, all Randall's struggling for breath and life, and suddenly boom, as if his spirit was singing his swan-song. That last evening his color had returned, his mind was clear, he didn't stammer, and his emotions were high and glowing."

Towers had entered. There was a perplexed, worried look upon his face as he listened to the words that continued to echo in the antechamber. Darrell explained the significance of those words. There were no chairs and he stood by the large open window that overlooked the entrance. Skinner was seated in an old wicker chair that looked like it had been around for a century.

There was a concerned tone in Towers' voice as he talked about his scheduled thoracoplasty with Darrell, who sat on the corner of the rectangular table by the window. He spoke in a soft confidential manner, as if he couldn't talk freely on the porch in the presence of Marrow and Blande, and Darrell was a compassionate listener. His cavity was located near or behind one of his bronchial tubes and Doctor Sheridan had told him that pneumos had failed to keep it closed and he was positive again after two years of rest. He was concerned because in a few rare cases where the resistance was low, TB had spread rapidly following the surgery and he had been told to take more exercise to build up his strength. He had visited several of the patients who had thoracoplasty. One was Patricia Brentwood who had a room down the corridor from the sunporch on the surgery ward. She had had the first stage, the removal of three ribs, and was scheduled for the second stage in three weeks. Towers hadn't signed the papers for his surgery yet. The thoughts of having a deformed, caved-in chest, and three stages of surgery was for him, a horrible decision to make.

That evening Darrell visited Patricia Brentwood. She talked in a very pleasant, soothing tone of voice as she described her rib surgery. There was still a wild glare in her light brown eyes from the shock of her last surgery almost two weeks ago. On her dresser stood a picture of her little girl; she was about three or four years of age, and little dimples backed her smile of tiny even teeth. Long curly hair streamed down in ringlets across her shoulders. Patricia Brentwood had the same smile and the same dimples, only a little more so. She was twenty-nine years of age and had spent the past two years here. She was a beautiful woman; the surgery hadn't taken her pleasant personality and beauty away.

"There's part of one of my ribs in the jar behind the portrait of Carol," she said.

Darrell examined the piece of rib, which was about four inches long.

"How many will you have to have taken out?" he asked.

"Nine," she replied, "three in each stage."

"It must be painful to have part of a rib cut out."

"That's the reason for the three stages of surgery. The thought is frightful, more so than the surgery. There are the after effects—the pain, the soreness, the discomfort, and the telltale scar. I will not wear the same style of evening gown or swimsuit. People will have to like me the way I am. That's life. After about a year and a half in here, my husband divorced me. My aunt is taking care of Carol."

"I lost my girl too," said Darrell. "I haven't seen her since I've been here. She does write once in awhile and she has promised to visit, but her parents will not permit her to see me. We were engaged to be married last June. But now, I can't really say that I blame her."

"Absence makes the heart grow fonder," she said with a laugh as she reached out for his hand.

Their hands touched tenderly and her grasp was firm in his.

"That's what they say, but certainly not for me."

Patricia Brentwood lay very still. Her eyes were veiled with a glistening film. Her light brown hair waved loosely upon the pillows and the shapeliness of her body was hidden beneath the covers. The delicate form of her breasts swelled the covers and there was a smile on her lips when she said, "Yes, but for whom? Not for me either."

The following day Towers was called to the office where he

signed the papers for his surgery, and that afternoon he was moved into the first private room, the one that Randall had occupied. It was across the hall from Patricia Brentwood's room. Doctor Sheridan performed the first stage of rib surgery early the next morning. Even though Towers was very sore, he appeared to be in good spirits. He had confidence in Doctor Sheridan and believed that thoracoplasty would do what pneumothorax had failed to do—keep the infected portion of his lung at rest.

Patricia Brentwood's second stage of rib surgery was delayed a week, since one of the local surgeons who assisted Doctor Sheridan was not available. She welcomed the additional time to build up her strength and she spent more time sitting up in bed. She enjoyed Darrell's company and he visited her frequently. There was a certain excitement and a restless, animated passion about him after the long siege of fluid. She liked his good looks and his youthful spirit. He was enthusiastic about the future and his plans for attaining the executive training program, he believed, were still achievable. Their discussions helped to keep him on a steady course and her courage inspired him as they talked of the future in a warm, heartfelt manner. This was her second attempt to achieve a cure. Her pneumothorax treatment had failed, for after she had been released four years ago, she said, "My husband made it next to impossible for me to get my rest. He didn't understand. He always wanted to go places and do things. We were both young and ambitious and then Carol came along, which was strenuous and made it more difficult for me to get the proper rest—something that men don't have to be concerned about, or at least my husband wasn't."

He enjoyed their brief visits. They talked more about the advantages and disadvantages of marriage for one who has had TB, and the problems encountered in keeping regular hours, a healthy diet, and the right amount of exercise. The evening before her scheduled surgery, she was feeling very low. She had expected a visit from her aunt. To brighten the evening and add some cheer, he brought over a small milk bottle with enough bourbon for two good drinks. Time passed swiftly with their talk about little things. They were laughing about milk bottles and bourbon that looked like ice tea when Mrs. Kenny entered to remind Darrell it was getting late. It was almost nine o'clock; time for lights out. Luckily, their glasses were empty, and if she suspected anything, she didn't let on. After wishing her the best in her surgery, he was forced to leave.

It was the latter part of September when Patricia Brentwood received her second stage of rib surgery. She maintained her pleasant disposition in spite of the pain and the soreness, which was worse now than the first stage.

At this time, Miss Sharen, who had been all thrilled with the thoughts and plans for her forthcoming marriage, left to join Doctor Harman in Toronto. He was soon to be assigned to the medical staff of the Royal Canadian Air Force, following a short training course. There was a high possibility that he might have to go to London and although she didn't like to be in London in wartime, she would go with him. Her cheerful care and encouraging words were greatly missed by the patients on the surgery ward. When Darrell couldn't eat solid food, she was instrumental in getting him a soft diet, including broth. For the past month he had prepared and ruled most of the patients' charts for her. Nurses' aides or trainees were now performing more and more of the nurses' duties.

Every tenth day, Bill Read, who had been released a month ago, returned to the sanatorium for pneumothorax, and he occasionally visited Darrell.

"It sure feels good to be out after almost three years. I was lucky to land a job, part time, at the Celina Style Shop. There's plenty of work now because of the manpower shortage and the war, but wait until you're released and watch the expression on their faces when you tell 'em that you can only work four hours a day. That always leads to a lot of questions and when you tell them why, most of 'em just politely tell you that they need someone full time. Most people are afraid of TB. They know very little about it and in the town of Celina, almost everyone makes it their business to find out where you've been and what you're doing. Why some of them will back up a step or two when they shake your hand."

Darrell laughed. "That's your imagination."

"It isn't my imagination when a person crosses the street, so he won't have to meet me."

"They don't understand and don't know how many tests were required prior to your release. I can see that it takes a lot of courage, patience, and determination to recover, and even more after a person is released."

"You're right. I've had negative sputum checks and cultures for a year now. The hay fever season is still on and even when I sneeze, it makes some people apprehensive."

"How long will you be required to take pneumos?"

"Five or six years."

"How's your father?"

"Doing fine. He's working full time in the cost department at the furniture factory. Are you still getting pneumos?"

Bill Read looked at his watch. "It's about time for lunch. I'm going to visit the gang at the new building. Maybe Maw and Pap Henry will invite me for lunch," remarked Read before Darrell could respond, and he asked again, "Are you still getting pneumos?"

"Every three weeks now and I can only take about 100 cc's of air. Since I had fluid, my lung is forcing its way out. That fluid really set me back. I feel lucky to get over the fluid as well as I did, and I'll be lucky if pneumos, with only 100 CC's of air, will keep my lung at rest, but who knows for how long?"

Another round of sputum checks were taken and Darrell awaited the results. He was also due for another X-ray. He had high hopes that his X-ray would show considerable improvement over his previous one, which had been taken three months ago. He hadn't heard a word from Pat Romane for some time. It was the last week of October, and the weather seemed to be waiting as colorful autumn leaves hung on the trees against a gray sky that seemed to never end.

Chapter XV

MISS DOWNLEY RESTS AT HOME WHILE PAT VISITS COLORADO AND ARIZONA

Darrell received his X-ray the first week of November. Several days later he was called to the office. As busy as Doctor Sheridan was, he took the time to personally review the patient's progress, and in most instances, he reviewed the results of the X-ray with each patient. His X-ray was clipped to the lighted screen and Doctor Sheridan announced, "The infiltration on your left lung hasn't cleared. It appears stationary and we believe it is. There hasn't been any change since your previous X-ray three months ago. The pleural wall on your right side has thickened with heavy calcification. We'll try to hold as much pneumo space as possible in order to keep your lung at rest. Your diaphragm is receding and your lung is sticking to the pleural wall at the base. We may have to give you a phrenic on your right side if your lung comes out."

There was a pause and Darrell asked, "What are my chances for getting well and staying well?"

"That's a big question. There are so many factors and so many variables. The statistics aren't good. Within the first two years more than fifty percent have a relapse. You have been fortunate, very fortunate. Many with less infection haven't done nearly as well. Your attitude is good, which is very important. I'm telling you this because you need to understand that recovery isn't easy. It's a long hard road and for most, a lonesome road. Your last culture and sputum check were negative. How long have you been negative?"

"Since May...May 21st ; almost six months. It has a special meaning. I waited a long time for that day."

"It'll raise you to class two, which permits you to walk to and from the clinic and you may discard your urinal. However, this doesn't mean that you can spend the afternoon or evenings visiting other patients. You must adhere to your classification as much as possible. How is your mother?"

The question surprised Darrell, but it wasn't noticeable.

"Fine. I've received several letters. As busy as Mother is, she manages to find time to write."

"Has the baby been born?"

"Mother's expecting the baby around the first week in December."

"And the family?"

"All right as far as I know. It was extremely difficult for the little ones and for Dad while Mother was here." He paused, thinking that perhaps Doctor Sheridan would comment about his mother's X-ray, and then continued, "Norma told me that the two little boys, they're in the first and second grades, would get hurt, either fighting with each other or playing, and then they'd come running into the house calling for Mother." Darrell laughed. "Well, Mother wasn't there. We call them Ike and Mike. They're always so full of tricks."

The doctor chuckled, then began in a serious tone. "It's extremely difficult for anyone who has to enter a sanatorium for any length of time. Your mother needed rest. She couldn't rest at home. People don't get the proper rest because their hours are irregular. I, myself, try to take an hour or two of rest in the afternoon, just like a machine that gets overheated, but the body isn't like a machine. An engine can be rebuilt or new parts added, but we can't add new lungs, and not for a long time to come. Therefore, you had better take care of the ones you have." The doctor paused, then added, "You had an appointment to the Naval Academy. Didn't you?"

"A first alternate appointment."

"All is not lost. Keep the good attitude."

Darrell thanked the doctor and walked slowly toward the sunporch thinking over the things that Doctor Sheridan had told him. More than fifty percent have a relapse within the first two years. It seemed incredible after years in a sanatorium. Why? What really happens? Adhere to your classification. He had just rounded the corridor leading to the surgery ward. Patricia Brentwood's room was directly ahead. He didn't feel the least bit sick. He was excited and happy, and some compelling urge made him stop, even though just a moment ago the doctor told him to adhere to his classification and don't spend time visiting the other patients. She was sitting up in bed and she knew that he awaited the results of his recent X-ray.

"I'm in class two," he said with a big elated smile.

She extended her arms to him. There was an exciting, happy gleam in her eyes. With a sudden impulse he leaned down and kissed her cheek.

"I feel happy too. I'm negative after more than two years." He kissed her lightly and fully upon the lips. "You deserve so much more. You're so invigorating."

Patricia Brentwood was scheduled for her third and final stage of rib surgery next week. She was slowly regaining her strength. Her color intensified as if life itself returned again after the shock of surgery had worn it away. Her eyes had a deep glowing sparkle filled with inviting loveliness. He held her hand with a warm touch of youth and beauty born of empathy of common misfortune and the passion of life. A life that for long months had been filled with thoughts and memories, that although wonderful, it wasn't really living, lying in bed alone waiting for surgery or for someone with the strength and health that had once been enjoyed to the fullest. Not a tear could change it, for youth and beauty moved on with all their impassioned, spirited feeling and magnificence. However, there came an appreciation for life and love and many things that had been taken for granted. Life flickered and with each pleasurable, precious heartbeat, youth was fleeting. Their visits, however brief, were filled with a desire and appreciation for an unknown, moving, secret life that was so near yet unattainable.

When Darrell entered the sunporch, Towers, who was scheduled for his second stage of rib surgery tomorrow, was trying to convince Marrow that he too needed thoracoplasty.

Doctor Sheridan had told Marrow that he wasn't able to take pneumos and that thoracoplasty was required. Marrow had talked it over with his wife and they had decided that there would be no cutting. It had something to do with their religion and Marrow was lying there growing weaker and weaker as the tubercle bacilli continued to feast as he wasted away.

"No sir," said Marrow, "that butcher isn't gonna cut my ribs out. Man wasn't made to be cut up like that."

"Damn," said Towers. "How can you say that?"

"I wanna keep my ribs."

"Doc will bring 'em back to you. You'll have short ribs."

"No sir! He won't get the chance. If I'm going to die, I wanna die in one piece."

"Damn," said Towers. "How can you say that? How can you be so narrow-minded? You're getting thinner and thinner. How much do you weigh?"

Marrow looked distressful. "I weigh 136. Three years ago I weighed 222 and not an ounce of fat."

Towers couldn't understand Marrow's attitude and he left the sunporch shaking his head. He could do no more to convince Marrow who had his mind firmly set against rib surgery.

Marrow turned his dark, distressful eyes upon Blande who had let out a bellowing cough.

When most patients received pneumos, their coughs lessened, but not so with Blande who continued to cough without covering his mouth as if to spite the fellows. They continued to relate gruesome stories about the happenings, mentioning the names of patients who had died and commenting with ridicule and irony whenever the black hearse drove up below the windows.

Blande opened his mouth wide and gave another whooping cough just as Doctor Sheridan entered the sunporch unexpectedly. It was late afternoon when he completed a review of the charts of the patients on the surgery ward. More beds were needed.

"Cover your mouth when you cough," commanded Sheridan. "We'll give you more air on your next pneumo. Maybe that will help."

Blande stared at the doctor, disdainfully.

Turning toward Marrow, the doctor said, "Your lung is sticking to your pleural wall." He said no more about thoracoplasty. It was most disheartening, but he respected his decision and as a last resort, as if to give Marrow time to consider, he added, "We have to give you a phrenic."

Darrell had told Skinner about his raise in class and as the doctor was about to leave, Skinner asked, "How about a raise in class?"

"How long have you been negative?"

"Since April; seven months!"

"Okay, but I want you to follow your classification. You've been here long enough to know what that means."

Skinner nodded his head with a big grin. He had asked at the right time and what a great feeling it was to get away from the commodes and Blande's loud coughs and unpleasant disposition just once in a while, if only to go to the bathroom. After he had hemorrhaged profusely, Doctor Sheridan gave him pneumos on both lungs to help heal his damaged lungs. Twice a week he had to go to the clinic where he was fluoroscoped and then he received about 500 cc's of air. He had stamina and youth was in his favor. His disposition, much like Darrell's, was one of willingness to do what was required with a determination to get well in spite of the unpleasant surroundings, whereas Blande was full of bitterness, as if everyone else was the cause of his being here.

Occasionally, Bunnigan stopped to visit on his return from the library, which was on the lower level in the middle of the southeast wing on the women's ward. The librarian was a kind middle-aged woman and a former patient. Every two weeks, or more often if requested, she would wheel the library cart through the wards for those patients who were bedfast. Bunnigan visited the library more frequently now, not to see the librarian who was rather strait-laced, but while on the women's ward it gave him a chance to visit with one of the women patients, a former nurse named Dorothy Marline who had worked at the sanatorium two years ago. He had become acquainted with her then. She had a slight infection that hadn't cleared with rest at home and had entered the sanatorium two months ago. From Dorothy Marline, Bunnigan had learned that Mary Jane Downley had decided not to enter the sanatorium. According to her doctor, her X-ray was somewhat better and it wasn't known what had caused the change in appearance of her X-ray. Perhaps it was caused by some stress or more likely a broken heart, for she was deeply in love with Doctor Herman. At any rate, Darrell was glad to hear that Mary Jane Downley didn't have to enter the sanatorium, but he was saddened to hear about Dorothy Marline, even though he didn't know her. According to Bunnigan, she would be up on exercise soon. She had worked at the sanatorium only one year, but during that time she had been heavily exposed to the dangers of the tubercle bacilli in her daily work. Two years later she broke down. She was one of the more fortunate ones whose infection had been discovered at an early stage as a result of regular physical examinations, a precaution and a requirement for the nurses.

One special characteristic of tuberculosis is that even an active disease does not usually cause noticeable symptoms until it is quite advanced, which makes screening tests more urgent and mandatory for anyone who has been exposed for a period of time.

Darrell admired the nurses for their dedicated services in view of the dangerous contact with persons with an active disease. It was a wonder that anyone would care to work in a place like this over a prolonged period of time when the exposure was so dangerous.

Bunnigan was in class seven, which permitted one half-hour of walking exercise, and he talked about going walking with Dorothy Marline. He participated in the weekly radio broadcast that was transmitted from the library. Records that had been loaned or donated by the patients and the women's club were played. The radio transmitting equipment had been built and donated to the sanatorium by a former patient. At this time Robbins was the announcer. The patients were beginning to take more interest in the program, and it was hoped that advancement made by medical research, in particular as it related to the treatment and control of TB, could be announced. However, progress was limited, but the hopes of the patients were high.

As Bunnigan left, carrying three library books, Skinner said, "I remember Dorothy Marline. She was a very lively, friendly nurse, a good looking blonde. Miss Downley has a nice slender, shapely figure, but you should see her."

Darrell's eyes sparkled. "I can hardly wait, for many reasons.

Do you realize that I've been lying here for nine months? What is there to do? Eat, read a little, listen to the radio, rest and sleep for twenty-four hours a day? We should get fat. I'm only 155 pounds and my normal weight should be 175. I could use some excitement and a better diet. Miss Sharen would see to it that I got seconds if I wanted. I sure miss her. Miss Barnes never seems to be around when we need her."

"You'll have to cultivate her," said Skinner.

"That will take some doing."

The following day, as scheduled, Towers received his second stage of rib surgery. For him, it was a sore painful day in his struggle to regain health. That afternoon a strong gale wailed through the partly opened windows of the sunporch, carrying with it icy particles of sleet. The beautiful autumn leaves were blown free and were battered and beaten by the sleet, and the trees of the wooded area that extended far to the south of the circular drive, stood there naked and cold, much the same as the patients in the old sanatorium as they waited for their treatment and surgery. As the afternoon rest hour approached, Darrell and Skinner opened all the windows of the sunporch and the sleet drifted along "Commodilly Row". With laughter, the fresh air addicts climbed into their beds and reached for their extra blankets.

"We'll freeze these bugs out if we can't get rid of them any other way," said Darrell as he pulled the blanket higher around his neck.

"Close those windows!" yelled Blande from behind the curtain.

"We'll freeze his ass off with the bugs," quipped Skinner.

"That wind will blow him through those cubbyhole doors," said Darrell.

Blande yelled again.

Marrow was laughing so hard that he had to hold his side.

"Hold it," shouted Darrell. "Just hold your horses. We'll fix the windows."

Miss Barnes who was seated at the nurses' desk just outside the glass paneled doors, finally arose and peered into the sunporch to find out what the shouting and laughing was all about. Then rushing in and nearly closing all the windows she said, "You fiends! You don't need that much air."

Then glancing at the drawn curtain she raised her nose higher and trying to hold a straight face, she left the sunporch shaking her head.

Transfusion didn't visit the fellows on the sunporch as frequently anymore. He didn't like Blande's attitude and he wasn't feeling as well as usual. Darrell stopped to chat with him from time to time. He continued to talk about the days of the depression, riding the slow freight trains and the rods when he couldn't find an open box car, and the places that he had been in his travels, but he wasn't himself. The effect of the long use of codeine was more pronounced.

Darrell continued to visit Patricia Brentwood. She waited anxiously for her third and final stage of rib surgery. Her outlook was good in spite of her broken home, and she continued to talk of her future when she would be released in a year or so.

He was also planning for the future, however silent, difficult, and uncertain. He was learning from the experiences of those that had gone this route before and were now on their second time around. His plans were in a state of flux as far as Pat was concerned, since she couldn't visit him and her letters were infrequent. It appeared that he would have to go it alone and plan accordingly.

Doctor Sheridan, at long last, did receive some help. Doctor Schmidt, a missionary doctor who recently returned from India, accepted a position as assistant surgeon. He wanted to learn more about the identification, treatment, and control of respiratory diseases and the latest techniques in chest surgery. His wife was a nurse and was appointed assistant superintendent of nurses to work with Mary Boswell and to learn more about the administrative duties. They had two daughters, twin honey-blondes, who were in their final year of nurses' training and both good looking. The family planned to return to India in about a year and continue his work there. Tuberculosis was rampant in India in the large population centers and medical care was inadequate.

Darrell was among the first to get a pneumo from Doctor Schmidt. He was an elderly Doctor with sandy hair, very kind and considerate. He pushed the needle between the ribs in a slow deliberate manner, then as the needle reached the pleural wall with its thickened, protective shield, it was suspended there in a slow, steady, piercing sensation and the sting was audible like the sharp snap of a banjo cord. However, under the guarded supervision of Doctor Sheridan, a more confident, swift, delicate, sensitive touch would come with experience. Almost ninety percent of the patients received pneumothorax treatment and some as often as once a week.

Doctor Schmidt assisted Doctor Sheridan in thoracic surgery. Patricia Brentwood, whose third and final stage of thoracoplasty had been delayed due to the shortage of surgeons, was the first surgery patient. She was selected because the risks were considered to be minimal and she was one of the most cooperative patients. After two lengthy rib surgeries, there developed a certain bond between the patient and the surgeon that only they could understand, for life was in his hands. The rib cage was further reduced by the removal of a part of three more ribs for a total of nine. A long incision extended from the back bone, just below and around the shoulder blade, to the side where the ribs had been cut, sliced and peeled away. As painful as it was, she accepted this operation in a good frame of mind, knowing that it was necessary and that it was the last.

Thanksgiving Day arrived. For most of the patients it wasn't a festive day, even though the customary turkey with dressing was served. It was usually a very special, festive occasion for the Darrell family, for it was their wedding anniversary. This year it was their twenty-fifth, but Joe could not be home and these were difficult times when everyone had to help. It was no time for festivity. The depression days were over, but not for the Darrell family.

The weather turned warmer again with an Indian summer. Darrell received a letter from Pat Romane. She was leaving by mid-December for a four-week vacation with her mother. They had reservations at the Broadmoor in Colorado Springs and at the Arizona Biltmore in Phoenix. Her father was a civilian flight instructor and couldn't get four weeks off, but he would join them in Arizona where some of the large Air Force flight training facilities were located. She had hoped to visit him before she left, but her parents wouldn't permit it. It was the same old story. Her parents insisted that the change in climate and the change in scenery would be good for her. She was all thrilled, and she would write and tell him more about it. He had hoped to see her during the Christmas Holidays, but then he wondered as he reflected on the summer when they had met...

"Summer, you old Indian Summer.
You're the tear that comes after
June times' laughter..."

By mid-December, Darrell, who had been in class two for a month, was raised to class three. He was now permitted to shave himself and he had full bathroom privileges. When he took his first shower in ten months, he turned the water on full force. Never had the water felt so invigorating, refreshing and vitalizing as he stood under the shower and let it pour and pour. But after the shower when he was stooping over to dry his legs, he felt a shortness of breath and his knees trembled. How weak he felt after ten months of bed rest and that long struggle with the fluid. He sat on the bench to regain a little strength before he took the slow walk to his bed. Never had he walked that slowly before. There were days on the farm when he walked all day behind a one horse cultivator through the long rows of tall corn. The extended time through the classes with more activity added was a necessary slow process for recovery.

On the sunporch in the fourth bed, Marrow, who had received a phrenic, complained about his stiff neck. He had a small incision about an inch and a half long at the base of the neck where the nerve that controlled one side of the diaphragm had been crushed. It kept one lung partially at rest for eight to twelve months until the crushed nerve became active again. It was an interim measure and could not replace the need for thoracoplasty, which Marrow had refused. Hopefully, it would give his lung time to heal. Marrow continued to complain and Blande continued his loud bellowing coughs.

Nevertheless, the patients awaited the approaching holidays, but for most there were no holidays. The tubercle bacilli took no holidays as these little parasites continued to feast. It meant a visit with the family, the faithful ones, and a few old friends who hadn't forgotten. They were the exception. They were the ones who had learned that a negative patient under treatment was not a threat to them. For some of the more fortunate few who had passed the tests, the negative cultures and sputum checks over a period of time, it meant a visit home for a day or two. For some others who had been long forgotten, there wasn't even a season's greeting card. Darrell received a letter and several cards from Colorado Springs and vicinity. Pat was learning to ice skate at the Broadmoor Ice Palace, and if she had a preference she would stay awhile, but they were leaving the day after Christmas for Arizona. Colorado Springs looking toward Pike's Peak with the Antlers Hotel in the foreground, and the Broadmoor nestled in the foothills of Cheyenne mountain against a red, purple sky were beautiful.

Darrell and Skinner received permission for an overnight visit home. The day before Christmas, he shaved and showered, and when rest hour was over, he dressed into his Air Force blue, flannel suit. He had time to spare and stopped to see Patricia Brentwood. She was resting comfortably, although very sore from her recent surgery.

"How handsome you look; really terrific."

"Thank you, I feel great," said Darrell as he approached her bed.

"I should never have had my surgery just before the holiday season, but I wanted to get it over."

He talked quietly and reassuringly with her before he had to take his leave.

As he passed Towers' room, he paused briefly to wish him a happy holiday season. Towers was doing well after his recent surgery.

Skinner was nervously pacing about and twice he had washed his face as he waited for his folks.

"You're going to wash the skin off your face if they don't get here soon," said Marrow.

They hadn't arrived when Norma and Charles came in, and Darrell left immediately with best wishes to all for the holiday season.

Chapter XVI

CHRISTMAS AT HOME

As the door closed, Darrell heaved a sigh of relief and took a deep breath of clean, refreshing air, leaving behind "Commodilly Row", his new friends, and all his saddened memories. The wintry, overcast sky seemed to be rushing toward him. The pebbles of the graveled drive slipped around beneath his shoes as he proceeded toward his '38 Chevy, accompanied by Norma and Charles, who was carrying his battered suitcase. There wasn't much in the suitcase, just a pair of pajamas, a change of underclothes, and a shirt. He really didn't need them for an overnight visit.

"Bet you would like to get behind the wheel again," said Charles.

"I sure would!"

Then he heard the words of Doctor Sheridan. "But, I'd better take it easy," he said. "Besides, Doc wouldn't give me permission if he saw me drive away and I don't want to take advantage of a good thing. I might want an overnight pass again."

"How is nurses' training?" he asked, holding the door for Norma.

"Oh, I like it, but I've had my share of bedpans."

He laughed as he seated himself beside her and closed the door.

The car started away with a loud rumbling roar. "The muffler blew out last week," commented Charles, "and I haven't had time to fix it yet, but your car runs swell and handles nice."

"How are things at home?"

"Same as always," answered Charles in a careless tone.

"You're not home enough to know," said Norma. "He's working in Lime now and since his draft number is coming up soon, he thinks he should have a good time before he leaves for the army."

"Sure, why shouldn't I?"

"That's the way all these young guys feel now. They don't care for anything else but the girls."

"You only live once."

"Did somebody tell you?" she bantered.

"For myself," added Charles, ignoring her sarcasm, "I don't mind going to the army. It's only when I think of the family..."

"How's Mother?" asked Joe, interrupting.

"She's fine," replied Norma.

"And the baby?"

"Big and healthy, weighed nine pounds when she was born. She's three weeks old. I guess Mother wrote and told you that they named her Francis Edwina. That's part of both their names. They wanted a boy."

"Ten girls!" exclaimed Charles, mopping his forehead.

"Yes, we're outnumbered, two to one," remarked Joe.

"Hey, watch where you're going," yelled Norma, "or let me drive!"

"I'd hate to spend Christmas in another hospital," said Joe and added with a chuckle, "I just came from one."

"Don't worry about my driving."

"As I was about to tell you," Norma continued, "We have all the arrangements made to have a family picture taken. This will probably be the last time that we're all home together for quite awhile."

"Will the picture be taken at home?"

"No, we'll have to go to the studio."

"Won't that be something!" said Charles. "I can just see old Barnett trying to keep the kids quiet."

Joe laughed. "It would be fun to watch if we didn't have to be in it."

The conversation continued and when they were driving through Celina, Joe remarked, "Celina looks pretty nice with all the Christmas decorations. Wonder what's going on in town?"

"Not a thing," replied Charles. "This town is dead."

"It looks good after being cooped up for ten months."

"So would any other town."

After several more miles, the car headed off the highway down a mile and a quarter stretch of gravel. Many a dark, wintry, icy night when the road had been covered with ice and snow, he had pedaled his bicycle over this road to basketball practice and games and once, when the team was playing out of town, he missed the bus. However, he caught a ride and arrived on time to get into his suit, but the coach didn't let him play the first half of the game. It had meant so much at the time. He was aware of some basketball scholarships, but because of financial conditions at home he couldn't arrange it. Those were happy days and now as he looked back, he realized that he could never play again. However, there would be other activities to compensate for active participation in sports.

They were approaching the huge cedars that formed an "L" along the northwest corner of the front yard, then into the driveway which separated the barnyard from the lawns bordering the house. It had been built of bricks by his grandfather, which he had hauled many miles by horse and wagon to the low rich land that he had cleared, tiled and drained.

As he stepped out of the car, the immensity of the graying sky and the open fields seemed to be closing in upon him.

"Where is Buster?"

"Didn't they tell you?" asked Norma. "Buster wasn't eating. He got so weak that he could hardly move, so they chloroformed him to put him out of his misery. He was almost fifteen."

Into his memory flashed the scenes of his boyhood days. Buster following him everywhere, always waiting for him, ready to play and run free as the wind in the wide open country.

The little ones rushed from the house, yelling and shouting, "Joe is home! Joe is home!"

Then into the house the noise and laughter continued. Ike and Mike stared at him curiously, as if he had risen from the dead. His mother showed him the new addition to the family, proudly holding her up.

"Look at your big brother."

The baby blinked her eyes and began to squall.

Just then, Mr. Darrell entered the kitchen with two geese that he had finished cleaning.

"These are the largest ones in the flock," he said, placing them on the table and added, "How does it feel to be home?"

"Feels great, except my eyes don't focus like they ought to."

"That's from staring at four walls all the time," commented Mr. Darrell, "and I imagine you do feel weak from lying in bed so long. When will you be released?"

"That will be another twelve months, which is the normal time for a test of health, strength, and recovery. It's a slow process to rebuild the body to a point where a person can live without the rigid routine of the sanatorium."

"Yes, I've heard the women talk about it, trying to stay well with all the outside activities," said his mother as she was preparing a shopping list of items needed for dinner tomorrow.

His father shook his head. "Some regimentation, twelve months, how lucky we are to be healthy."

"Yes, I took too much for granted. I never gave it much of a thought before," he said and then asked his mother, "Are you going to make dressing?"

"Yes, Daddy or Charles will have to go to town. I don't have enough English walnuts for the dressing. Those old black walnuts we have are too strong."

"This goose is much fatter than the other," said Mr. Darrell. "The meat will be more tender and juicy."

In the corner the three little tots were holding hands and jumping around in a circle singing, "We'll have a goose for Christmas...a goose for Christmas..."

"Since we only have the one roasting oven, I'll roast the fat one and fry most of the other that I can't get in the oven," said Mrs. Darrell.

"A fat goose for Christmas...a fat goose for Christmas..."

"Will you be quiet? I can't hear myself think!" said Mrs. Darrell, "and Joe doesn't want to hear your chatter."

Mrs. Darrell handed the shopping list to her husband.

"Want to come along Joe?"

"The drive has been enough for me for one day. I guess I'd better rest. I'm not use to so much activity."

"Can we go? Can we go?" cried the little tots.

"If Daddy will take you," said Mrs. Darrell, happy to have them out of the house for a little while.

After the scramble for hats and coats, the house became quieter and Joe seated himself in the old rocker while his mother began to prepare the evening meal. They talked over things in general at the sanatorium.

"What did Doctor Sheridan say about my leaving?"

"Never mentioned a word about it, although he did ask

about you when we had a talk about my last X-ray. He said that you needed rest."

"Doctor Hattery said that I never had TB and that I shouldn't have been there. Norma wants me to go to the hospital where she is training for a check-up. I'll go when the baby is a little older, just to be on the safe side. You know how it is after you've been over there."

"Well don't worry about it. I would trust Doctor Hattery."

"I'm so busy. I don't think about it."

Charles entered. "How soon are we going to eat?"

"Soon as Daddy gets back from town," she answered. "He hasn't changed, Joe. He's always ready to eat."

Charles gave a big grin as he looked over his mother's shoulder to see what she was cooking.

"Are you going somewhere tonight?" she asked.

"I'm gonna see Katy."

"We want to have Christmas for the little ones tonight."

"Everything has been arranged," he replied.

"Maybe Joe wants to use the car?"

"I don't have anywhere to go. I just want to enjoy being home."

"Maybe you'd like to lie down for a while, Joe. We fixed a bed for you in the far front room, so you won't have to climb the stairs."

"I feel fine. I had two hours of sleep this afternoon."

Charles left the room to join the girls and help with the Christmas decorations. Mrs. Darrell laughed. "They've got something planned for tonight. The girls are in the living room decorating the cedar tree that Daddy brought from the woods yesterday. They have to lock the doors to keep the little ones out. Only the three smallest ones believe in Santa Claus."

At eight-thirty that evening, the family gathered around the tree in the living room. All the lights were out except those on the tree and on the holly wreaths in the windows when in walked Santa dressed in a red and white suit. His eyebrows were white as snow and he wore a long white beard that covered his mouth. He chuckled as he mumbled a few words with Ike and Mike who made a grab for his beard or his nose that was very red, as red as lipstick. Santa cuffed Ike alongside the ear almost knocking him down. Then Mike started to pull at the seat of his pants. The rest of the family was bursting with laughter and Mr. Darrell had to call them off Santa.

Santa set down the huge sack that he was still holding and with a chuckle and a "ho-ho-ho" now and then, he began to distribute the packages—first to the little ones; a present for each. Their eyes bulged as they hurriedly pulled away the wrappings. There were shoes and socks and other items of clothing. Ike and Mike didn't like their presents. They each had a suit of long underwear. Ike held up his suit, making fun of the open flap in the back, while Mike took a swing at Santa. But Santa gave them two more presents that contained some shoes, which they liked and really needed. All the younger members of the family were showing and comparing their presents. Joe hadn't been able to bring any gifts. He received two pairs of pajamas, one red and one blue in a paisley design, which were surely needed.

There was fruit, nuts, and a few chocolate drops for everyone, that is, if they ate sparingly. Richard, who was about eleven years old, was stuffing himself with chocolate drops when Mrs. Darrell said, "Don't make a pig of yourself. Save some for the little ones."

"The little pigs," laughed Richard, grabbing another handful.

"Richard," shouted Mr. Darrell, "do I have to get the strap on Christmas Eve?"

Santa patted his tummy and waved good-bye.

The older members of the family were talking of the Christmases of the past.

"Twenty-one years ago tomorrow, at nine P.M.," said Mrs. Darrell, "Joe was born; a big, twelve-pound baby boy. He was a real Christmas present."

"Some big Christmas present," injected Mary.

"The doctor wanted to use instruments, but my mother wouldn't let him. After all the effort, what a thrill it was to hear him cry when the doctor spanked him. It was a cold wintry day with a lot of snow. We lived just a half-mile down the road in the house that Daddy built. We called it our bungalow and that's where Joe was born."

The door opened. Katy entered followed by Charles. There was still a smudge of lipstick on his nose. Soon Mary's boyfriend arrived, followed in a short while by Ruth's boyfriend. While the fellows waited for the girls, they compared draft numbers. Charles' number was nearest the top of the list and as the discussion continued, Joe excused himself and retired to bed. It was shortly after nine o'clock and way past his bedtime.

His thoughts drifted. He was thinking of the holidays a year ago. The night when the champagne glasses clinked as they lay in front of the huge fireplace in Pat's living room. Their elbows crossed and after the first sip, her eyes glowed and sparkled when she saw the ring in the bottom of the glass. They embraced with long smoldering kisses. What a night it was, with such fond memories and pleasant dreams.

The floors that had been littered with nutshells and the wrappings of presents, were clean, but there was the evidence of Christmas day. Mary and Ruth served the Christmas goose, delightful and wholesome with all the trimmings, at the large dining room table, reserved for special occasions, where fourteen members of the family were gathered around. Mr. Darrell was seated at one end of the table between the two tricksters, Ike and Mike. And Mrs. Darrell was seated at the opposite end between the two smallest girls, then the bigger children and the middle-sized ones to fill in, and fill in they did. It was a happy family get-together in spite of the hard times and Joe's troubles, and it was the last for quite some time.

After the Christmas dinner, the house was put in order and took on a much quieter air, and the tree, though jostled about for two days, stood serene and shiny as the gaiety of Christmas subsided. The eldest girls helped to get the little ones washed and neatly dressed in their Sunday best, and then the family piled into the family car, a '39 Chevy, and into Joe's old '38, and drove to the photographer's studio in Celina, about three miles from home. Surprisingly, the little ones were well-behaved and followed the photographer's instructions. Mr. and Mrs. Darrell were seated on each side of the front row. Mrs. Darrell held the newborn baby on her lap while the younger children stood in the front row and the taller ones in a row behind them, fifteen children in all. Later the picture was shown on the front page of one of the church papers published in Cincinnati, Ohio.

After the picture had been taken, and without any further celebration, Joe was on his return trip to the sanatorium. His battered suitcase contained an added change of under clothing, several shirts, and socks and pants, since he expected to take outdoor exercise by springtime. In addition to the neatly wrapped package with the two pair of pajamas was a pint of bourbon, a present from Charles with best wishes for "A Happy Birthday, A Merry Christmas, and A Happy New Year".

Chapter XVII

NEW YEAR'S EVE

When Darrell returned, a group of Christmas carolers were singing below the windows of the old ivy-walled sanatorium in the cold gray twilight. They were a welcomed sight, for even though some of the patients may have been forgotten, it gave them a feeling that someone cared. The choral group sang the joyful hymns in a soft, soothing, pleasant chorus as they slowly made their way around the sanatorium with frequent stops below the windows where some of the patients had gathered. For most of the patients it helped to brighten a rather sedate Christmas day. There had been few visitors for the old lungers, and for the newer patients there was the fear of the unknown brought about by the limited knowledge of the disease itself and the stigma that had been attached to it.

New Year's Eve arrived with all the sad, bitter memories of the past year that could not be easily forgotten. Darrell, who was wearing his red paisley pajamas and his long blue robe, walked slowly through the darkened corridor. It was so very quiet on the surgery ward. There was an eerie effect where the light reflected from the partly opened doors. When he arrived at Patricia Brentwood's room, she was reading a magazine. She was lying flat on her back with her head propped against the pillows as best she could so that she could read. The lamp added a lustrous effect to her light brown hair and her light blue pajamas.

He greeted her with a, "Happy New Year."

"Happy New Year. I'm so glad you came!"

She extended her hand to him with a smile. That wild glare from her last surgery was noticeable.

"Did you have a nice Christmas?" he asked, taking her hand.

"I had a very quiet Christmas. I could only see Carol for a few minutes and I didn't feel well. As you know my last surgery was terrible. I'm glad it's over. I would have given anything to be home at this time of the year. How was your visit home?"

"Very enjoyable and very quiet. There wasn't any Christmas cheer. Dad and Mother don't drink. Oh, maybe a glass of beer or wine on special occasions, but seldom anything stronger."

"There wasn't any here either."

With a happy, mischievous smile and a twinkle in his eyes, he raised the pint of bourbon that had been hidden in the deep pocket of his robe. "Let's drink a toast to '43. May it be good to both of us."

"Wonderful! I'll drink to that. There's some ice water in the pitcher and there's another glass on the dresser," she said as he was looking about, and continued, "It was so nice of you to think of me on New Year's Eve. I was feeling very blue trying to drown my thoughts in a magazine."

"I think I'll ask Doctor Sheridan to transfer me to the new building. I've been in class three for two weeks."

"But you'll have to be in class five."

"I know, but I'm sick and tired of that sunporch."

"Don't rush it. You've waited this long and I'd miss you."

"And you'll be moving to the women's ward soon and then I

couldn't see you until I'm up in class," he said, and as their eyes met, he leaned down and kissed her. It was wonderful and so inviting.

"More likely I'll be moved next week," she said, and added, "Have a good reason when you ask Doctor Sheridan."

"It will be better for me at the new building. Let's drink a toast to Doctor Sheridan."

As he poured another round of drinks and put the bottle away, approaching footsteps could be heard in the corridor.

"He is a good doctor and surgeon," she said as their glasses clinked.

The footsteps drew nearer, slapping the floor hurriedly and then stopped momentarily. The night nurse, Miss Klingland, teased in surprise as she was about to enter. "Mr. Darrell!" she exclaimed with one eye crossed at him, "what are you doing here?"

"Happy New Year!"

"You'll have a Happy New Year if Doc finds out!" she said as she proceeded to adjust the windows for the night.

"But you wouldn't say anything," pleaded Patricia Brentwood. "Not tonight."

"It's after visiting hours. I'll pretend that I didn't see him." Then turning toward Darrell, she added, "On one condition—that you leave by nine."

Then she spotted the extra glasses. "What are you..."

"Happy New Year!" he said, interrupting.

Her shoes slapped the floor as she walked over, raised the glass and sniffed, then her eyes crossed as she raised them out of the glass and looked at him. "Where is it?"

"Where's your glass?"

She gave a deep raspy laugh. "I'm on duty! Wait until I get off duty." Then she turned and throwing her long legs loose jointedly, she left the room.

He shrugged his shoulders. "I tried. Can't win 'em all."

"She'll be back," said Patricia Brentwood with a smile. She was feeling better. "Miss Klingland goes off duty at nine tonight."

It was almost nine o'clock. She reached for his hand. The touch was warm as his fingers played along her arm and her lips were soft and thrilling as his lingered upon hers, enraptured by all the ecstasy of life that they shared. A good understanding friend here added a special touch along life's troubled way which meant so much to both of them.

Approaching footsteps alerted them of Miss Klingland's return. She appeared holding a small paper cup. He filled it with bourbon. "Happy New Year," she said, raising her cup, and with a wink and a blink, it was dry. Then she drank a cup of ice water and after the exchange of greetings, he poured another round.

"It's nine o'clock. I'm off duty and I've got a hot date tonight."

"I could say something there," he said raising his glass.

"Here's to it and here's from it, and here's back to it again. If you're to it and can't do it, you may never get back to it to do it again."

She laughed. "I could do something there, but I won't. Not tonight," she said with a wink as she left the room.

When he returned to the sunporch, Blande's radio was blaring with an early New Year celebration and Skinner had his radio tuned to another channel. He soon fell into a heavy sleep and slept through the ringing in of the new year. He was awakened about seven o'clock by a shoving and tugging at his arm as Miss Barnes was taking the pulses and temperatures. The stench along "Commodilly Row" came like the rising tide and lingered there. It was bath day for Blande and Marrow, and therefore the windows couldn't be opened. Blande complained and coughed more than ever without covering his mouth and Marrow, his face thinner now, looked sternly at Blande with dark wrinkled brows. Marrow continued to protest vehemently against surgery of any kind, as he complained about a stiff neck and the shortness of breath.

Several days later when Joe stopped to see Patricia Brentwood, she told him that she was to be transferred to the women's ward today. Their visits had been wonderful. He would miss her.

"I'll most likely be in one of the sunrooms, because everything is so crowded. I hate to think about it after the privacy."

"After I'm transferred to the new building, I'll come to visit you when I'm permitted to go to the library or to the weekly broadcast. I haven't had a chance to talk to Doc about the new building. He hasn't made his rounds recently."

"Perhaps you had better go to the office to see him."

That afternoon, after the rest hour, she was moved to the far southeast sunroom, the one where his mother had been. He talked to Miss Barnes about the new building and learned that Doctor Sheridan was in surgery. She sensed his restlessness and asked him to rule some charts for her. He gladly accepted to show appreciation for her thoughtful care and her change in attitude toward him. Perhaps it was also a change in his attitude. He wasn't really aware of any change, but there was a better understanding of what the nurses really did for each of the patients that impressed him most; their unselfish devotion to their profession with all the associated risks. While she was explaining how she wanted the charts to be ruled, there was a heavy scent of smoke.

"Something's burning," she said, sniffing the air.

As Miss Barnes hurried into the corridor, he slipped into his shoes and followed the nurse around the corridor to the right. She had entered the third cubbyhole. This was the older section of the sanatorium. A gray curtain of smoke clouded the room and then, as she was pushing and half carrying a little elderly man into the corridor, the room seemed to burst into flames. He was so weak or dizzy that he could hardly stand. He was clad only in a surgical gown and coughed heavily from the smoke as he leaned against the wall. Darrell remembered that there was a fire extinguisher hanging along the corridor by the drug room. Miss Barnes was returning with several pitchers of ice water from the adjoining rooms when he returned with the fire extinguisher. The smoke was thicker now and the flames more intense. Skinner and two other patients who awaited surgery, brought more pitchers and a bucket of water. Together they were able to contain the fire and get it under control. When they were searching for the cause of the fire, they discovered that a quart bottle of whiskey had spilled, plus the evidence of the cigarette burns in the bedding and the smoldering hole in the mattress.

"I couldn't understand why the fire had spread so fast. The cause, all that whiskey," she said, shaking her head. "I'm sure thankful that you thought of getting the fire extinguisher when you did." As she put her arm around his shoulder and held him closely, he was tempted to kiss her, but she turned quickly away toward the little elderly man who was sitting on the windowsill.

The following afternoon while Darrell was returning from the bathroom, he saw the same little elderly man paddling along in his bare feet, skinny legs, and a bare behind, as he was clad only in the surgical gown. He disappeared around the corner of corridor where Miss Barnes spotted him and hustled him back to his bed.

"I wanna smoke," he said.

"I'll smoke you! You don't run through the halls without your pants," said Miss Barnes who had him raised so that his feet barely touched the floor as she hurried him along. "You press the button when you want a nurse and we'll bring you a cigarette."

When Darrell returned to the sunporch, he told Skinner

about his decision to ask Sheridan to be transferred, and that was all they talked about for the remainder of that day and on into the following day. Then when it became evident that Doctor Sheridan wasn't going to make his morning rounds, Darrell decided to go to the office. He preferred to go alone, but Skinner went along with him. The office door stood ajar. Darrell knocked without hesitating at the sound of voices within.

"Come in," answered Doctor Sheridan, who was reading and discussing the X-ray films upon the lighted screens with Doctor Putner, the surgeon from Michigan who had cut Darrell's adhesions.

"Well, what brings you two to the office?"

"We would like to be moved to the new building," replied Darrell.

Sheridan laughed and turned to Putner who was eyeing them curiously. "Here's a couple fellows who had one foot in purgatory," he said, and there was a pause while he studied them. "Why? Is there anything wrong?"

"You know how it is on the sunporch," answered Darrell.

"With the commodes we can't open the windows as much as we would like and the coughing, well it gets on a fellow's nerves after awhile."

"What class are you in?"

"Three."

"And you Skinner?"

"Four."

"Do you think you're ready for the new building?"

They nodded their heads.

"It's different at the new building," he continued. "You'll have to get up for your meals and you'll have to make your own beds."

The fellows continued to nod their heads. They could think of nothing else no matter what the chances might have been.

They were aware of the routine and the conditions at the new building, and Bunnigan had informed Darrell that there were several beds available. Their request was made at an opportune time.

Doctor Sheridan was in need of more beds on the surgery ward and he knew there were three beds vacant at the new building.

"Darrell, I'll raise you to class four, but you'll have to remain in bed as much as possible for the next month. By now I believe you realize how important it is and what the risks are. It's like you have one lung to go."

Darrell beamed with happiness as he promised that he would.

"And you also, Skinner," added Sheridan.

They left the office, smiling at each other with elated thoughts. That evening they bid farewell to the old patients on the surgery ward. Towers awaited his third stage of rib surgery. Transfusion was little more than a bag of bones, but he could still chuckle and with a laugh he said, "There isn't enough meat on my arms for the nurse to stick me with the needle. She's sticking me in the legs now. I'm still waiting for that shot that will give me a cure."

"I'll stop by to see you once in awhile. So long for now old pal," said Darrell. But deep within Darrell knew that it wouldn't arrive in time.

Shortly after eleven the following morning, they alighted from the old elevator on the ground floor level. The cold crisp air took their breath away and they pulled their coats tightly about them, blinking and squinting their eyes in the sunlight that reflected from the crusted snow like moles from their cavern. With each step, the crunch, crunch of the snow was like laughter to their ears, taking them farther away from "Commodilly Row," and a healthier environment.

The door of the new building opened into a passageway that led to the lobby where a large round table covered with huge potted ferns of various species stood beneath a center skylight. The bright light reflected on two of the four beige walls and in the illuminated corner was an old victrola containing many old records. Next to it stood an upright player piano with rolls and rolls of old recordings on its top, and to the right in the opposite corner, grew several large rubber plants that took away the appearance and odor associated with hospitals. Along the far wall were several leather armchairs and a settee.

Maw Henry made her appearance from the kitchen located on the east side of the passageway.

"Paul Skinner," she said, extending her arms in welcome as she approached, "I'm glad to see you."

Skinner bobbed his head and added a devilish, though happy grin. This was his second tour, so to speak, after almost three years since he was released.

"And you're Mr. Darrell, aren't you?" she added as she shifted her dark sparkling eyes upon him and without waiting for him to answer, her eyes shifted again to Skinner.

"We have rules here as you already know," she continued in her high-pitched voice, studying them intently and waving her arms. "The east side is completely filled."

As she led the way toward the west side, they passed through two swinging doors where eight low beds lined the wall, four on each side that faced the west windows overlooking the small artificial lake. Scattered about were four fellows, idly chatting.

"The last bed on the right will be yours, Paul, and that is your locker in the corner beside it," said Maw, and turning to Darrell, she added, "The second bed on the left will be yours." Then pointing to two dressers that stood in the middle along the west wall she continued, "You'll find two vacant drawers there."

With a hurried glance about, she started for the doors where she turned saying, "I'll have to check my charts before I can tell you what your bath times are."

"So you finally made it!" exclaimed Bunnigan.

"It's been a long, long struggle, but better late than never. I'm lucky to be here, if you know what I mean. It was touch and go for awhile," he replied jokingly as he proceeded toward the three lockers that divided the windows in the left section of the long dormitory.

"You'll like the west side. We don't get the morning sun, but there's a good gang of fellows on this side. We had a lot of fun on the sunporch, but it's livelier here. There are three or four older fellows on the other side. You wouldn't like it. They are very serious-minded and want everything quiet. When they get on this side, the old fellows don't last long before they want to be transferred."

With a chuckle, Darrell removed his topcoat and hung it in the middle locker that he found to be vacant. "I'm sure I'll like it here. The sunporch was getting unbearable. Blande's coughing was driving me up the walls."

"We hardly ever hear a cough here."

"That's incredible for a group of old lungers."

"This is Higgins," continued Bunnigan. "He has the bed between us."

Darrell shook hands with Higgins, a red-faced fellow with a toothless grin who carried one shoulder two inches higher than the other; the one that he favored after his rib surgery.

"And that's Millford," nodded Bunnigan, "who has never told the truth since he's been here."

Millford, a short guy with straight black hair plastered to his scalp, arose with a laugh. He looked young for his age and he had rib surgery on his right side. "If I told the truth around here, they'd know me better than I know myself."

Amid the guffaw that followed, they shook hands. Then Darrell removed his suit coat.

A short wiry fellow with blonde curly hair, who Darrell had met before at the clinic while they waited to have their fluid drawn off, was walking in a sidling manner toward the swinging doors "It's time to eat," yelled Blake as he passed through the doors.

When they entered the lobby, a line had already formed and they proceeded to the bathroom to wash their hands, then joined the queue.

In the kitchen Pap Henry, a quiet guy with graying hair, was dishing up the plates with a boiled dinner of potatoes, cabbage, and beef, while Maw set the small dishes of custard and half pints of milk on the counter. After Darrell received his food and was about to leave the counter, Pap Henry said, "You're a big fellow and look as if you could use another helping. You may come back for seconds."

Darrell thanked him and then joined the fellows at the west table where Higgins was cutting his beef very fine, or attempting to. "The beef looks good. Is it tough?" he asked Higgins who was munching a small piece.

Higgins wrinkled his red face in a grin and was about to speak when Bunnigan asked, "Higgins, when are you getting your teeth?"

"My gums have to shrink," he replied, squinting his eyes and looking about.

"Shrink?" exclaimed Millford, "the dentist slapped mine in two days after he pulled them. "How about you, Barton?"
Barton, a middle-aged fellow, neat in appearance, was laughing silently and nodded his heed.

"Yeah, Millford," replied Higgins, "you had this jerker who wanted to collect his money in a hurry from the board."

"Oh no I didn't. I got 'em just before I entered three years ago...cost me thirty bucks."

"Thirty bucks!" shouted Higgins, dropping his fork. "I have to pay eighty."

Amazing, thought Darrell, these guys aren't more than thirty or thirty-five and already they have false teeth.

"Darrell, you have a good even set of teeth," continued Higgins. "What did you pay?"

"The teeth are all my own and I intend to keep them."

They were all laughing except Shorty Anderson, a black fellow who sat at the end of the table shaking his head. "You're lucky to have eighty bucks."

"His wife's paying for 'em," taunted Millford.

Higgins' face reddened. "My insurance helps to support her."

"Insurance!" exclaimed Shorty, his fork poised at his mouth.

"Insurance from the oil company where he use to work," added Millford. "And they were glad to get rid of him."

Higgins' face grew redder still and he was about to shout when he saw Maw approaching.

Maw set her stern eyes upon them. "You're making much too much noise. Doesn't do any of you any good to get so excited. A fine example you are to the new patients." There was a pause as she looked about. "Take the example of Mr. Barton," she added. A slight smile crossed Barton's face as Bunnigan almost choked and Higgins and Millford bowed their heads to keep from splitting their sides with laughter.

After dinner when the fellows were preparing for rest hour, Bunnigan who was taking off his pants at the south corner of the dormitory remarked, "Barton, you sure have Maw fooled...Ho, ho-o. Take the example of Barton...Ho, ho-o."

"Remember the day that he moved in?" added Millford.

"Maw said to us, 'My isn't he a gentleman, so polite and cultured.'"

"How's the budding romance with the big blonde nurse?" asked Bunnigan.

Barton smiled but said nothing as he climbed into the first bed to the right of the swinging doors. This was Barton's second time in. He had heavy infiltration in both lungs. He smoked heavily and was short of breath, and according to him, he had never raised any positive sputum. Barton's wife had died of tuberculosis about two years ago. They had been fairly wealthy, but the long illness cut heavily into the profits of his business. He was from a small town in the north central part of the state where he had operated a plumber's shop and wholesale business.

For most of the patients in the new building, it was the beginning of a new way of life after months of bed rest, and it was the beginning of the test of exercise to determine if they were able to return to a normal life completely arrested and free from any active TB. For the more fortunate ones, like Shorty Anderson, who had discovered their infection early through the Army physical, the test wasn't as severe as it was for Darrell whose disease was moderately advanced when he entered. And there were the unfortunate ones, like Towers, who had to return to the old sanatorium to begin again. However, where there was life there was hope. The percentage of those who made it in the 1940's, if known by the patients, would have been discouraging, for nearly twenty-five percent of those admitted died in the sanatoriums, and of those released, fifty percent were dead within five years. It wasn't a bright future for Darrell. It was more necessary than ever for Darrell to heed Doctor Sheridan's words and to follow the intent of the classifications, as difficult as it might be or become when one is feeling well and others are at play.

A letter and a greeting card arrived from Pat Romane, showing the Arizona Biltmore with Squaw Peak and the desert in the background. She described the beautiful grounds, the groves of oranges and grapefruit, so colorful and loaded with fruit in January. There were German prisoners of war taking care of some of the grounds. What an ideal place, she wrote, at this time of the year. The weather was ideal too, in the seventies during the day and the nights were cool. She was trying to get a good suntan before she had to return and she was enjoying the horseback riding, tennis and swimming.

That evening he wrote a lengthy letter to Pat with the good news about his transfer to the new building, the procedures, the surroundings and his new friends. He also wrote about his visit home for Christmas and he hoped that she could visit him soon. Now that he would soon be able to take some exercise, it would be good to get away for a short while. They could go driving together, walking, and dancing.

Chapter XVIII

SPRING ARRIVES

Maw Henry ran the new building like a battleship. She had silver-gray hair that was always set in perfect waves and her voice was high, like that of a canary. Pap Henry was a quiet sort of a fellow, easy going, never ruffled, who took his orders from Maw without a word in return. Rest hours were observed the same time as in the old sanatorium. Breakfast was served promptly at seven. The beds had to be made whenever they were not occupied. Every Tuesday and Friday the bed linens were changed, and then the sheets had to be neatly tucked in and the corners square like hospital beds. Maw and Pap Henry took Friday evenings off and usually did not return until late Saturday. Occasionally, on Friday nights when there was no one around, the fellows on the west side celebrated. However, with the words of Doctor Sheridan in mind, Darrell and Skinner remained in their beds and tried to follow their classification as much as possible.

Once a month regular sputum checks and cultures were taken. A positive report would strike with the force of lightning, sending the poor unfortunate victim back to the old building, as had happened to Towers who had received his second stage of ribs and awaited his third. Skinner walked to the clinic for his pneumos every week and for Darrell, it was every tenth day. The fellows who were required to take outdoor exercise seldom left the building as January continued with its cold, nasty wind. They were waiting for spring to arrive with its balmy breezes.

February came. Darrell was raised to class five. The fellows became tired of seeing him lying in bed and reading throughout the day, but he was intent on following the class five level.

"Is he going to stay in bed forever?" asked Barton.

"You'd think that he came here to get well," replied Millford.

"We'll fix him," added Bunnigan. "Come on Higgins, give us a hand."

The four wheeled Darrell and the bed into the lobby alongside the huge potted ferns where they left him. He remained there about an hour. The fellows from the east side had a big laugh whenever they passed, but Darrell didn't mind. He was enjoying the joke and the new west side initiation procedures.

"What does this mean?" asked Maw when she returned from the office and spotted him.

"It must be part of the new initiation for the west side."

"Who pushed this bed out here?"

"I certainly didn't. I'm only in class five. I want to tell you how nice this winter garden of potted ferns and those rubber trees are. I was admiring them."

"But, you can't stay here. You'll ruin my flowers," she said in pompous tones as if he would contaminate them. And as if she were about to flap her wings and fly, she added, "Get up and I'll help you."

She walked along with her hand on the head end of the bed as Darrell pushed. When she opened the swinging doors, laughter rang loud and long. Maw looked about sternly, but said nothing as she left the room while Darrell replugged his bedlamp.

Late that Friday night when Darrell was half asleep, Bunnigan approached. "Want some ice cream?"

"Sure," he said as he climbed out of bed.

In the next bed Higgins was sound asleep and his radio was blaring away. And in the dimly lit lobby, Millford was picking the lock on the wide upper half of the Dutch door next to the kitchen counter. By trade, Millford was a baker and a short order cook until he was committed to the sanatorium about three years ago. Since then he had received thoracoplasty on his right side. He was nervous and quick mannered, and smoked about two and a half packs of cigarettes a day. A cigarette hung from the corner of his mouth as he continued to work the lock. When the upper half door opened, Bunnigan gave him a boast. He climbed through and opened the door, which entered the kitchen from the passageway. The lower half of the Dutch door required a key to unlock the dead bolt. In the kitchen they moved about hurriedly—each scrambling three eggs.

"Where's the bread?" asked Darrell.

"Maybe you'd like a glass of beer too," replied Millford.

"I just came for ice cream, but how would you like a shot of bourbon?"

There was a knock on the door. For a moment the three looked at each other.

"Caught like a rat in a trap," whispered Darrell.

"Open the door!" sounded Barton's voice. "It's me."

Barton entered followed by Skinner.

"Damn!" said Millford with a mouth full of eggs. "May as well wake up all the fellows!"

"Why not?" taunted Bunnigan. "They won't kick us all out! Will they?"

"Who cares?" said Barton, breaking the eggs with one hand. "I'm ready."

"You may be ready, but I just arrived," said Darrell with a laugh. "I'm just beginning to start on my exercise and I've got to be able to earn a living when I'm released. I'll probably have to spend the summer and most of next winter here."

Barton laughed quietly as he scrambled the eggs with a fork. He had a high forehead and his brown curly hair was beginning to thin. He and Miss Barnes had been secretly meeting several times a month, but the word was beginning to get around. "This is better then the old building and a fellow can manage to get away once in awhile."

"Darrell, you'll make it out," said Bunnigan. "Don't worry."

"I'm not worried. If we just have our health and a good environment, we'll all make it out. Doc said, 'Adhere to the classes. You have one lung to go.' I feel much better since I've been at the new building. Did anyone wake up Blake and Shorty?"

"I'll wake 'em up!" said Skinner.

"Just the west side. Those East lungers wouldn't appreciate it and they would only get us into trouble," said Millford.

Darrell dug into the five-gallon container of ice cream. "Say, doesn't Maw miss the ice cream? And who takes the blame for this?"

Barton flipped his eggs onto a plate. "I overheard Maw tell Miss Barnes that she shouldn't give out so much ice cream and when Miss Barnes replied that she didn't, Maw was flabbergasted and dumbfounded."

"How is she?" asked Bunnigan.

"We're lucky to have Miss Barnes on Maw and Pap's night off. She really does all she can for us and she never says a word about our raids on the kitchen," said Barton as he finished his eggs.

Darrell had finished one dish of ice cream and offered to serve Bunnigan and Barton. "She was very strict with us on the surgery ward and wouldn't stand for any nonsense."

Barton handed his dish to Darrell, saying, "She can be tough when she wants to be."

"You should know," bantered Millford.

"What a build she has!" exclaimed Bunnigan. "Does she give you a good ride?"

Barton laughed with a snicker.

"He won't laugh if Doc catches him," gibed Millford.

"Or if Beetle gets wise to him," added Bunnigan.

Skinner returned followed by Blake and Shorty Anderson, who was blinking his dark eyes under the bright light.

"Higgins was sound asleep," said Skinner, "and his radio was blaring. He just grumbled and rolled over on his side."

Blake talked in a curt style as he brushed his blonde hair with his hand. "Skinner flashed the overhead lights."

Seven excited fellows hurried and scurried, bumping into each other as the last of them tore into the ice cream with laughter. Shorty Anderson moved faster than any of them.

"This ice cream is real yummy," said Skinner.

"Never did ice cream taste so good," said Darrell.

"We better get this place cleaned up and get the hell out of here," said Barton as he finished his ice cream.

"Why?" queried Darrell. "There's no one around. You don't suppose Beetle would be around at this hour?"

Bunnigan glanced at the kitchen blinds that had been drawn. "Weasel-face might have seen the lights on the west side from his cottage across the lake."

"I'll keep a lookout," said Darrell, leaving the room.

After the dishes were piled in the sink, washed and dried, and the kitchen put in order, Millford and Bunnigan made the final inspection. And ducking, almost crawling for fear that Beetle might spot their movement, they re-entered the west side through the swinging doors.

"There isn't a sign of Beetle or anyone else around,"

announced Darrell.

"I'm not the least bit sleepy," remarked Bunnigan. "Let's play some poker."

"Good idea," answered Barton. "We can sleep tomorrow."

"Where'll we play?" asked Blake.

"In the corner of the lobby," replied Millford. "The light can't be seen from there."

"You going to play, Darrell?" queried Bunnigan.

"Not tonight."

"How about you Skinner?"

"Yeah, I'll play."

"That'll make a five-handed game," added Barton. "Let's go."

Shorty didn't play poker but prepared to watch as the five gamblers settled down for a long session. Darrell turned off Higgins' radio and the room became very quiet. He soon fell asleep. When the fellows returned to their beds from the poker session, it was after four in the morning.

Three hours later as a cold gray dawn was beginning to break and Miss Barnes was taking the pulses, she announced, "Well, you guys had another party last night."

There were a few snickers, but no one commented. The telltale pulse rates of the poker players were significantly higher. It was only Barton's influence that prevented her from turning in a report and the charted pulse rates were adjusted so that there was little noticeable change recorded. Occasionally, in the early evening and sometimes under the cover of night, Barton slipped out to meet Miss Barnes. She had a room at the nurses' building, just around the circular drive from the men's building.

And so the parties continued, but in a much more subdued manner. March arrived; Darrell was now in class six, which permitted him to be up about an hour and a half a day. Another round of sputum checks was taken. There was one positive report. Maw spoke very little that day and the gloomy atmosphere was noticeable. The fellows on the east side moped around spending more time than usual in their beds. When evening came and Skinner tuned in his radio, he picked up the weekly broadcast of the amateur station that originated from the library of the sanatorium.

"Say Darrell, since we're in class six, we're allowed to attend those broadcasts."

"Yes, I plan to go next week. I had my quota of exercise for today. What goes on at the broadcast?"

"They just play records," replied Millford from the bed on Darrell's right.

"What does Bunnigan do?" queried Darrell.

"He calls himself the chief engineer," said Skinner.

"Chief engineer...Ha!" added Millford. "He just goes over to meet the women who are up in class. He's got a romance started with some blonde. She was a nurse here two years ago; Dorothy Marline."

"Wonder who will be the new announcer after tonight?" asked Skinner.

"Perhaps Bunnigan will," remarked Darrell.

"He couldn't play with the women then," added Millford.

"Robbins did all right as an announcer. He really took an interest in the broadcasts."

"Yeah," remarked Skinner shaking his head. "He's really had tough luck. After more than six years he finally gets to class eleven and then he gets a positive report."

"What's Doc say about it?" asked Darrell.

"Doc told him that he needed thoracoplasty," answered Millford, and added, "Tomorrow he'll be transferred to the old building."

"He won't take ribs though. That's why Doc gave him a

paraffin pack," said Darrell thoughtfully, and added, "Will he take them now?"

"No," answered Skinner. "He said that he didn't want a scar on his back for the rest of his life."

"That's what Maw told him," remarked Millford. "He was one of her model patients from the east side, so she's taking it pretty hard."

"I can understand why Maw is taking it pretty hard," said Darrell. "This is Robbins' third time around and the thoughts of rib surgery can be frightening. However, it's better to have the scar if that's what it takes to recover. How's Towers doing?"

"He had his last stage of ribs weeks ago, but he hasn't had a negative sputum check yet and that has him worried," said Millford, who had gone through three stages of rib surgery.

"That's one thing that will break a fellow faster than anything else. Towers doesn't show it, but he does worry and he likes to cover up by pouring it on somebody else. I don't know Robbins very well, but I'd bet that's what caused him to break down, his worrying. Why you hardly ever see him around very much and he was in class eleven, afraid to take a walk. Exercise in accordance with the classes is an important part of regaining health."

The positive report was indeed a catastrophe for Robbins. With his head bowed and a paleness upon his face, he left the east side to begin the saddened, doleful walk back to the old building. His mind was set not to accept thoracoplasty though the fellows had tried to convince him that it was the thing to do. But who could tell him any differently unless they themselves were in that position and faced with the decision to make?

Bunnigan, who was now in class twelve, had developed a sudden interest in outdoor exercise. Even on the cold wintry afternoons, he would put on his galoshes and follow along the path that led around the lake into a wooded area. Then it became evident that the romance grew stronger and when the afternoon rest hours were over, he would watch the north windows until he saw her walking slowly on the drive that wound its way along the barren hedges and away from the confining walls. As she disappeared around the first bend, he would follow.

"There he goes with his nose to the trail," commented Blake with laughter one afternoon when the snow was blowing so that Bunnigan's figure was hardly visible.

"I ran into them one afternoon at the corner store," added Millford. "They had bought some cheese crackers and were feeding each other like two love birds." Millford went through the hand to mouth motions. "One for you...one for me...the old guy who runs the store threatened to run them out if they didn't stop their cooing like two love-sick doves."

Blake laughed loudly, showing the slight gap between his two front teeth. "What happened to your girl, Millford?"

"She was a released couple of months ago," and he added a chuckle, then said, "I got a letter from her the other day. All that was in it was a three-cent stamp."

The guffaw followed.

"Thought you were going to get married," added Blake.

"Him? Get married?" exclaimed Barton. "Of all the stories he can tell."

More guffaw followed.

"Do you still have her ring?" asked Blake curtly.

"Yeah, here it is," he chuckled. "I ought to send it to her."

"Wouldn't you rather give it to her?" asked Darrell.

"That isn't all he'd like to give her," commented Barton.

Darrell was concerned. He hadn't heard from Pat for quite sometime, since her vacation in Arizona. He had written several letters that had gone unanswered. There was a telephone in the hall entrance which was part of Maw and Pap's living quarters, but no long distance calls could be made from there nor could the patients make any local calls.

That afternoon when Bunnigan returned from his afternoon walk, Maw glared at him as the rest of the fellows had already been served. Pap said nothing and served Bunnigan.

"You'd better watch out," said Barton. "Maw will put the Weasel on your trail."

"I know," said Bunnigan, and turning toward Darrell, he asked, "Do you know who will be at the broadcast tonight?"

Darrell thought that Bunnigan was referring to Patricia Brentwood.

"Dorothy told me today that Betty Gordon had asked about you."

That evening, all the fellows from the west side went to the broadcast. The program consisted of recordings and Blake filled in as the announcer. There was only a small selection of records, most of which had been donated by the patients. The transmitting equipment was a homemade affair built by a former patient. As for the studio, there was the musty smell of old books on the library shelves. Only one portion of the books were in use and the others were covered with dust. Bunnigan was the self-appointed chief engineer and after adjusting and tuning the volume, he was free to help Dorothy Marline, a shapely blonde who took charge of changing the records. As Blake didn't care to be the announcer, the fellows began to take turns, which added to the merry mix-up of everyone selecting a record of his or her choice. Blake was devoting much of his attention to Phyliss Carlyle, an attractive, tall slender brunette. There were ten women seated around the edge of the library, all happy to be up and share in the activities. Darrell was looking through the small selection of records with Betty Gordon. She had a fascinating way about her as she laughed and talked with Darrell. Last summer, when she was in class eleven, she had a relapse and was now in class eight on her way up again. She selected a recording that reminded her of last September and the long quiet walks along the lake not far from here. Then she had to drop back in class and begin that long, sad, disappointing and lonesome recovery through the series of classes. One September night, more than three years ago, they had danced to the tune.

She handed him the record saying, "Play this one for me, Joe."

He announced the tune as, "September Love Song, dedicated to a lost memory and to youth, beauty and health wherever they may be. The carefree, handsome youth burning with love and the innocent, soft, tender, sweet, loving beauty searching for love and health."

"...The leaves of brown came tumbling down, remember, last September, in the rain..."

Darrell and Betty began to dance. Bunnigan and Dorothy joined them, like lovers in a close embrace. The dancing added to the gaiety. It was good exercise, but dancing wasn't permitted.

After the broadcast, Darrell stopped to visit Patricia Brentwood.

"Thought you might be at the broadcast," he said.

"I'm only in class three and I hope to be in class four in another month. I enjoyed the broadcast. It was better than usual. The September Love Song introduction was nice. You have a good radio voice—really sounds pleasant. You should be the announcer."

"Thank you. Later perhaps. It would be better if we could get the broadcast studio transferred to the men's building. It's much more pleasant there. The library smells rather musty."

The sunroom was crowded. Another bed had been added since his mother had been there. He recognized two of the women and they inquired about his mother and the baby. He talked briefly about his visit home and told them that Mother would have an X-ray taken next month at Dayton where his sister, Norma, was in nurses' training. Nine o'clock was approaching and the women were getting dolled up. It did give them a lift and helped to make them feel better, even though they weren't going anywhere and there were no visitors expected. For some it had been years of the same routine, but looking their best enhanced their mental disposition which was so vital to their well-being.

When Darrell returned to the men's building, Bunnigan and Blake, who had gone walking with Dorothy and Phyliss, were still out. It was after ten when they returned. Spring was in the air. Mr. Beetle was also on the lookout. He made a note of their late return, however nothing was said.

The following week, Higgins went to town to get his teeth. The night of the weekly broadcast, all the fellows from the west side were there except Higgins. It was a rather quiet evening. Miss Bellhaven, a strict elderly nurse, was there to supervise. There was no dancing. The word had apparently gotten around, for now they had a chaperone. Darrell and Betty planned to meet on the next day in the afternoon.

Chapter XIX

A WILD PARTY

The lights burned until after nine that Friday night on the west side of the new building. When Bunnigan entered, the fellows were still preparing for bed. He cussed loudly and banged his locker. His face was red, reflecting thoughts of concern. Wearing a slight grin, he approached Darrell who had just crawled into bed.

"Beetle caught us," he whispered and added a sly laugh.

Darrell looked as if he didn't believe what he had just heard. "What did he say?"

Bunnigan laughed and his face grew redder still. "We've been kicked out. The son-of-a-bitch wanted us to pack tonight."

"Both of you? Dorothy too?"

"What happened?" asked Millford from the bed next to Darrell.

"We were just caught out too late. The son-of-a-bitch was laying for us."

"What are you going to do?" asked Darrell.

"I'll talk to Sheridan tomorrow."

"You only had another month to go," commented Darrell, "but what about Dorothy?"

"Five weeks. I've been in class twelve almost two months and she expected to be released in about seven weeks."

"Maybe Beetle needs the beds. The place is getting more crowded. I heard Pap say that Beetle would like to put two more beds in here."

A hush prevailed. Then a few comments were exchanged followed by laughter at Bunnigan's expense.

"Where's Higgins?" asked Bunnigan.

"He's still out after his teeth," answered Darrell sleepily.

Most of the fellows were sound asleep when Higgins entered shortly after eleven and flashed the overhead lights. He stood just inside the doors grinning from ear to ear and showing his sparkling white teeth.

"You damn fool!" shouted Millford. "Turn off the bright lights."

"Look what I've brought for you dogs!" he exclaimed, pulling out two fifths of bourbon.

Then Higgins walked to the foot of Barton's bed. "My, isn't he a gentleman."

Barton was snoring and Higgins jarred his bed. He reared up, blinking his eyes and stared at Higgins who was holding the bourbon at the foot of the bed.

At that instant, Millford snapped off the lights.

"Okay you dogs, if you don't want a drink..."

"Pull the shades," commanded Barton as he turned on his bed lamp.

"Yeah," said Darrell, "we don't want the Weasel on our tails." And he began to chuckle, "Bunnigan got caught tonight."

"The hell!" exclaimed Higgins with bulging eyes and began to laugh.

"Uncork that bottle," said Bunnigan as he began to draw the

shades. "It may be funny now and tomorrow will take care of itself."

"This is the time to celebrate," added Darrell. "There's nothing more that we can do now."

Higgins grinned showing two sets of teeth.

"He'll still be showing them tomorrow when Miss Barnes comes in," bantered Blake in curt tones.

"With these choppers, I can bite the cork off."

"Hey Shorty," shouted Higgins as the fellows were bringing their glasses, "get over here. There'll be no sleeping tonight."

"Come on Shorty," said Bunnigan. "It may be the last chance. Tomorrow I'll be on my way."

Shorty Anderson had been a teacher in one of the local schools. He taught the second grade plus a course entitled, "Introduction to Physical Education" which consisted mainly of gymnastic drills. He was to be released as soon as he received the report of his X-ray.

After two drinks, Barton and Darrell began to sing:

"You are my sunshine, my only sunshine,
you make me happy when skies are gray...
You'll never know dear how much I love you.
Please don't take my sunshine away..."

Shorty stretched like a cat. His black eyes and face were hardly visible in the dim light as he rolled out of bed, then handed his glass to Higgins who had begun to pour another round.

"Higgins, are you ever going to use your right arm?" asked Millford, who was still a little worried about his own thoracoplasty side after a fall down the ravine. He had fallen two weeks ago when he was walking by the way of a shortcut to the Alpine, a road house, two miles away by the highway or less than a mile by the shortcut.

Higgins grinned from ear to ear as he continued to pour the drinks. He was in his glory tonight. He was proud of his choppers and his thoracoplasty that he had received on his right side about a year ago. He was in class twelve and although he had only two months to go before he was to be released, he was afraid to move his right arm.

"Shorty, you need another drink," said Higgins, "and you other dogs can pour your own."

With two good drinks, Shorty became talkative. "You know, those guys on the east side are afraid of their own shadow. What will they do when they get out? I don't know what I'm going to do. I'll only be allowed to work four hours a day. Doctor Sheridan said no competitive sports and no gymnastics. I liked wrestling and track and the school board don't want me to teach anymore. They said I'd infect their children. I only had a little spot on my X-ray. I shudder when I think of the cavities you guys had." After another drink, he continued, "When I stopped at the draft board for my classification card, or rather a reissued one, the gal says to me in her smart nasty tone, 'You got TB.' And I asked her what that was. Then she growled and snapped, 'You got tubercossis...tubercossis, you hear?' I thought it was something like syphilis the way she sneered in that nasty tone. I never could say it and neither could she. I thought it was hereditary, but the county health doctor said that was all wrong and that the schools needed better courses in health education...anyway, I like sports and wrestling."

"Say, speaking of sports, let's go to town," shouted Millford. "I know a good sporting house."

"I'd like to see Shorty operate," commented Higgins, jokingly.

Bunnigan, a diabetic, was nursing his second drink. "I'll go for the fun of it. I'd like to see Shorty operate."

Blake laughed. "Can you take another piece so soon after your evening walk?"

"That's one way to get in your daily exercise," commented

Darrell. "Someone said that a good piece of tail is like a ten mile walk."

Skinner flipped the ashes off his cigar as if he were sitting on top of the world. "I could use a piece of tail."

"Why you squirt," jeered Bunnigan, "a good piece of tail would kill you."

"They won't let him in," laughed Blake.

Skinner took a deep drag, then blurted, "The hell they won't, burp-bah."

"We're all going then," said Millford, taking it for granted.

Darrell laughed. "Everybody's going for the fun of it, the excitement of life, and sexual intercourse."

Barton poured another drink, then held it high while he sang, and one by one the others joined in.

"...The other night dear as I lay sleeping,
I dreamt I held you in my arms.
And when I awoke dear, I was mistaken.
Please don't take my sunshine away..."

"Who's gonna call the cab?" asked Blake, and then he laughed loudly showing the gap between his front teeth.

"I know one of the drivers who knows the hospital grounds," announced Millford.

"So do I," added Barton.

Frequently on Friday nights Barton would walk to the corner where Miss Barnes would meet him in a cab.

"How's the blonde?" asked Bunnigan.

Barton snickered and began to pour another round of drinks.

"Poor Miss Barnes," said Darrell, "Maw and Pap still think that she's eating all the ice cream."

Higgins yawned. "Maw says that she's gaining too much weight."

"Look at that!" bantered Darrell, "Higgins doesn't have any wisdom teeth."

"What? No wisdom teeth?" shouted Millford. "And he paid eighty bucks!"

"Oh, my hell!" churned Skinner, blowing out a puff of cigar smoke. "No wisdom teeth!"

Bunnigan shook his heed. "That dentist really rooked you."

Millford was serious. "You aren't going to let that dentist get away with eighty bucks that easy, are you?"

Barton winked. "Better go back to town next week and see that he makes it right, the jerker." Then he began to sing again:

"You are my sunshine, my only sunshine..."

"I'll call the cab," said Millford, leaving the room. There was a phone in the reception hall in the front between Maw and Pap's rooms, but the patients weren't permitted to use it.

While he was gone, Blake discovered that the bulb of his bed lamp was burned out, and just as he was finished unscrewing Millford's bulb and proceeding to replace it with his own, Millford returned.

He immediately saw what had taken place and flew into Blake with a roundhouse swing to the side of the head. Blake dropped the bulb on the bed and returned the swing. More blows were exchanged. The two were evenly matched. Blake's pajamas were ripped off his back. Then he grabbed the collar of Millford's pajamas and tugged away, dragging Millford with them. Both of them kept swinging their fists wildly. The pajamas tore with a ripping sound and the crescent-shaped scar of Millford's rib surgery, cut neatly below his sunken shoulder blade, was clearly visible.

"How crazy can they be? Is that what bourbon does to them?" asked Darrell. "After all the time that they have spent here and all they've been through, to fight and risk tearing their heeled lungs apart. We've got to stop them."

"Let them fight it out," said Barton as Darrell started to separate them.

Blake threw Millford's pajama top at his face and the chase started. The chair that stood near them spun about and crashed against the wall. As the chase continued the chairs that stood in a line were knocked wildly about until Blake fell against the wall by his bed.

There Darrell and Bunnigan separated them, but they were no more than separated when the fight began again. They ended up on Higgins' bed with Higgins underneath them, and taking several blows in his attempt to get away.

Barton strode back and forth as he rolled his eyes with a mean stare. "I'm a mean son-of-a-bitch. I choke 'em until their tongues hang out and then I hang 'em by their tongues."

That didn't sound like Barton at all. For a moment Darrell thought that he had gone off the deep end. He was so serious, then suddenly he began to laugh, a long deep laugh.

"I'm a lover, not a fighter," said Darrell, who had his share of fights when he was growing up. At one time he was about to enter the golden gloves tournament, but after several stiff jabs in the nose, he decided against it. He didn't want his face battered and disfigured.

Darrell and Bunnigan pulled Blake and Millford off of Higgins, and Shorty brushed his hands as if to indicate that he had stopped the fight. Blake and Millford panted for breath like two wild animals and glared at each other with wildfire in their eyes.

"That's our trip to town," said Higgins.

Slowly Millford turned away, then picked up his light bulb from his bed. "I didn't get to call the cab; the phone isn't working."

It was after four. The bourbon was finished and the lights were turned out. As Miss Barnes took the morning pulses, she announced, "I see you fellows had quite a party."

"Bunnigan and Shorty will be going home soon, maybe

today," said Barton. "You know how it is—a little celebration."

"It was more than a little celebration by the beat of these pulses."

Barton snickered. "Bunnigan was caught last night with Dorothy Marline."

"Oh, no! Not her! I hope her husband doesn't hear about it."

Shorty closed his eyes and rolled his woolly head from side to side. "Oh, my head," he moaned.

That morning Miss Barnes watched as the fellows from the west side ate sparingly, except for Bunnigan and Darrell who did their best to eat a complete breakfast to keep up their nourishment. When breakfast was finished, Bunnigan left immediately to see Doctor Sheridan. He wasn't in the office. This was Saturday. Bunnigan went to his residence; a large house located about a hundred feet from the office. Bunnigan had hoped that he could talk to Sheridan before he received Mr. Beetle's report. Together, they went to the office to review his record. The doctor had already received a report of last night's escapade. There was no alternative. The rules had to be obeyed. He had to maintain order and respect. Bunnigan was fortunate, because his health wasn't in jeopardy. He had been negative for sixteen months. However, the doctor cautioned him that as soon as his phrenic nerve began to innervate the diaphragm on the arrested lung, he would need another phrenic. With Doctor Sheridan's permission, he called his wife from the office.

She came that afternoon at three. Bunnigan already had his bag packed and when she appeared, he shouted good-bye to the fellows as if it was well-planned and nothing had happened. She only smiled in her quiet manner and appeared very happy.

It was a dismal afternoon with low overhanging clouds. Betty and Darrell met for their half-hour walk. It felt good to be out and away from the four confining walls, the medicinal odors, and the watchful eyes. Out of sight of the hospital, they walked hand in hand.

"This is great to get away for a walk," said Betty. "Do you know that it has been seven months since I had that one positive check. Doc says that I won't have to spend as much time in each of the classes now."

"It is great," said Darrell. "This is my first walking exercise after thirteen months."

"The sunroom is crowded and I'm tired of listening to the same four women. Sometimes I think the walls are talking. There are no secrets."

"What have you heard about Dorothy?"

"The women were shocked!" she said. "They had Bunnigan practically raping her on the cement; the cold cement by the elevator. Dorothy is afraid that her husband will hear about it. She said that Doc agreed to keep their love affair secret. It was only a passing fancy, something to do to pass the time. Her husband came for her during rest hour. Can you imagine—Beetle wouldn't let her stay until Sunday, not one more day, after all she had done for the patients here two years ago. That was before Doctor Sheridan was here."

"Beetle has forgotten what it's like to be young and to live again after months of forced rest in the same old room. He does a lot of snooping around. It's a wonder someone hasn't hit him over the head."

"He deserves it, but don't get any ideas."

A long, low whistle of a slow freight train could be heard in the distance. "Maybe a freight train will hit him," said Darrell with a laugh. "We'll have to be careful and adhere to the rules. It is easy to forget and overstay the time limit when one is walking and enjoying it." He was thinking of the future when they would be able to take longer walks, deeper into the wooded area that bordered the golf course and the lake.

The following morning when Maw entered to take the pulses, she was in a light and airy mood. Perhaps it was the weather, or perhaps it was the fact that Bunnigan was gone.

"Good morning! Good morning!" she chirped. "Get up you little scal-li-wags. Rise and see the sun," she continued to chirp in a high-pitched voice. And as she was about to leave, she said, "You all keep your sputum cups for a check tomorrow morning."

Shorty obtained his release, and that week Doctor Sheridan told Darrell that since he was on exercise, he was losing his pneumo space, but that he would try to hold it as long as possible and then give him a phrenic.

Darrell's brother Charles, and Katy, made a surprise visit later that week, just prior to his induction into the armed services. As the afternoon rest hour was over, they went for a drive through the back country. Charles offered him the wheel. He enjoyed driving his car again and prior to his return they stopped at the Alpine. It was a small, clean, road house with a long bar and a small dance floor with a jukebox to one side surrounded by tables. At that time of the afternoon there were only a few customers. They ordered three bottles of beer and Charles told him that Mother's X-ray, which had been taken at Good Samaritan Hospital where Norma was in nurses' training, was all right—not a sign or trace of any infection.

Late that afternoon when Darrell had returned to the new building, Doctor Sheridan made one of his unexpected visits. Carefully, he checked the charts at the nurses' desk in the lobby accompanied by Mary Boswell and Miss Barnes. And when they entered the west side, Higgins was grinning from ear to ear.

"How do you like your teeth?" asked Sheridan.

"Doc, I don't have any wisdom teeth."

Doctor Sheridan shook his head unbelievingly. "No wisdom teeth!" And he turned his head and winked.

Mary Boswell and Miss Barnes exchanged glances, trying to hold straight faces.

"I don't think that you'll need wisdom teeth," added Sheridan.

"But, Millford and Barton have wisdom teeth on theirs."

The fellows roared with laughter.

As the doctor turned to leave, he winked again, then asked, "Where's Blake?"

"He's taking his walk," replied Darrell.

"What do you suppose he wants with Blake?" queried Millford after the doctor and nurses had left.

"By the sound of his voice, I would say it wasn't good," commented Darrell.

"We're lucky our rapid pulses aren't recorded on Saturday mornings," said Barton.

Blake returned from his walk in time for the evening meal. He was in a happy mood and continued to sing:

"...Oh, the Indian arrows used to fly,
like raindrops through the sky,
deep in the heart of Texas..."

"Doc was looking for you," said Darrell.

"Yeah, what for?"

"He didn't say."

The following Monday morning Blake was called to the office. There, Doc gave him the report of a positive culture and also, a positive report on his last sputum check. He returned in a sullen mood and silently began to pack his bag for the long, lost trudge to the old building.

"What did Doc say?" asked Darrell.

"I can't take pneumos and my phrenic isn't doing enough good since I'm on exercise. My fluid messed me around," continued Blake in his terse tones. "I'm scheduled for thoracoplasty," he said in a broken voice and there were tears in his eyes.

Darrell accompanied Blake on his slow walk to the old sanatorium, as if there might be some way to help. Blake thought that perhaps his fight with Millford may have caused his breakdown that resulted in the positive sputum check. However, there was a previous culture, which was also positive. Darrell tried to reassure him that it was coincidental and that there were other factors involved. Darrell got off the elevator on the first floor and Blake proceeded to the second floor surgery ward where he had been assigned to a private room.

Darrell went to the library and then he visited Patricia Brentwood who was now in class five and would soon be able to attend the weekly broadcasts. The glowing sparkle of her light brown eyes was deeper now as she talked about the other classifications and the summertime. In her voice the courage and determination were evident, even after two and one-half years.

The beds at the new building were all occupied as soon as they became vacant, or by the following day. Three fellows in their mid-twenties now occupied the beds vacated by Blake, Anderson, and Bunnigan. And on the east side, two fellows in their late teens recently moved in and were named for certain outstanding characteristics, such as "Elsie the Cow," for the one who drank a lot of milk, usually two pints at every meal and one in between meals, and "Nabisco Kid," for the one who always seemed to be eating crackers in bed. They were all the more fortunate victims who had discovered their infection early as a result of the Armed Services screening program. With the arrival of the new victims, the games changed also. Although Poker predominated, some of the other games introduced were: Bridge, Hearts, Casino, Five Hundred, Euchre, Chess, Checkers, and Dominoes. The games changed with the desire to do something different. Darrell enjoyed all the games. He was lucky in Poker. With the arrival of the younger patients, there was more of a gambling spirit, a more carefree mood, and the ante was raised. Even though he was more than eighty dollars ahead, he preferred Bridge to Poker. But for some, no games could satisfy them. They cared less for reading and didn't take the required amount of walking exercise, which was so important toward regaining strength in preparation for their release. They tuned in to the ball games on the radio and waited for their wife or a friend to go for a drive, or to go to a tavern or home, if they lived near enough. But most of the old patients didn't have many visitors. They were almost forgotten except for their immediate families. Darrell's brother Charles was in the army, and in the springtime on the farm his father and mother were busy with their daily work, providing the necessities of life. Sunday was suppose to be a day of rest, but not so with a large family to provide for. His sister, Mary, came to see him once in awhile and brought several of the newer, popular recordings that he had requested, most of which made the hit parade on the weekly broadcast.

Darrell became the announcer and Betty Gordon assisted with the selection and the changing of records. The equipment and studio were transferred to the lobby of the new building where the surroundings were more pleasant. It gave the women patients, who were in class six or higher, a chance to get out of the old building on Friday evenings and to meet others. And it gave the fellows an opportunity to escort the women back to the old building and to go for an evening walk when the weather was favorable. High on their hit parade at that time where such records as:

"...missed the Saturday dance;
heard they crowded the floor;
Don't get around much anymore..."
And,
"I'm going back to where I come from...
where the honeysuckle smells so sweet
in the lilac bush."

Another tune played frequently by popular request, which really livened up the place and almost jarred the bedfast patients out of their beds, was a Spike Jones recording:

"Pass the biscuits, Mirandi;
pass them and kiss me goodbye..."

The broadcast became a fun session. The popularity increased and more and more of the patients participated.

By the first of April, Darrell was in class seven and Betty Gordon, who had been raised in class every two weeks, was in eight. Following the broadcast they went for short walks whenever time permitted. With a restraint of emotions they returned to their confining rooms by the nine o'clock curfew hour. The outdoor exercise was limited by the amount of time that class seven permitted, and he tried to stay within that limit—one half hour. They met occasionally following the afternoon rest hour when they were permitted to go walking. It was wonderful to be able to get away for a short walk and they enjoyed their brief meetings. Their minds were open to their limitations as they exchanged thoughts and experiences, and she was understanding since she had had a relapse last summer after a year and a half spent here. They were going to be more careful now and live each day as it came along and enjoy life to the fullest extent possible. The little things and health meant so much now. They didn't feel that two old lungers should get married for they couldn't properly support themselves, and if a family came along and one should have a break down, it would be extremely difficult for the other. They were willing to face life as it was, but why should one expose herself or himself to greater danger or risks than he or she already had. They talked freely of their experiences. In the relatively short period of time that he had been there, he had seen too many romances that ended unhappily because of health. She talked about her engagement, which was broken when she had her relapse, but not forgotten. He was in the Air Force and she hoped that they might get together again when he returned.

As they became more acquainted, he told her about his love for Pat Romane and their engagement, and that he hoped her parents would permit her to visit him. He hadn't heard from her for some time.

"Why didn't she answer?" he asked.

"Out of sight; out of mind," said Betty.

He wrote a brief letter to Pat with best wishes for her upcoming twenty-first birthday and their engagement anniversary date, both on June tenth. Even though it was the first week of April, he had to hear from her and his letter included the following heartfelt requests: "Answer me, my love. Please tell me when we will meet again. You'll never know what my heart is dreaming of. Please answer me, my love."

Chapter XX

A NIGHT OUT WITH PAT ROMANE

The third week in April, Darrell received a letter from Pat Romane; she planned to visit him the last Friday in May, about eight-thirty in the evening. This was the day when her parents planned to be away. She had finally received her parents' permission to buy a car, but a good car of any kind was hard to find since almost all production of automobiles stopped shortly after war had been declared. She would be driving her mother's 1940 green Ford. It seemed strange that she hadn't mentioned a word about the special letter that he had sent for her twenty-first birthday and their engagement anniversary, both of which were on the tenth of June.

Pat arrived early. The broadcast was over. He was ready and waiting by the north windows of the west side when she drove into the parking lot and he hurried to meet her. As he entered the passenger side, she said, "You're looking good, as handsome as always and you have gained some weight."

He looked at her as if he couldn't believe that she was real. It had been such a long time-more than fourteen months. He held back the tears as he said, "You are even more beautiful than I remember."

Tender lips met with a yearning, burning love and from deep within, a tingling sensation surged to the touch of their lips.

"Would you like to drive?"

"Very much," he exclaimed as he proceeded around the front of the car. Then he asked, "Have you eaten?"

"Yes, before I left."

As he drove away from the sanatorium, a huge fiery sun was descending behind a slightly clouded sky. "That's a beautiful sunset," he said. "What a brilliant glow."

"It reminds me of the sunsets in Arizona, almost all the colors of the rainbow—the various shades of red, pink, orange, violet and blue."

They were driving west over the back roads that led to the Blue Note, and she was all excited and talked about her visit to Colorado and Arizona. When they entered the Blue Note, the place was deserted except for a couple of lovers in the far corner. The bartender looked at them as they proceeded to a table near the small dance floor, then ordered two champagne cocktails.

When they were served, he offered a toast, "To your twenty first birthday."

"Oh! You are a month early!"

"I know. We need to take advantage of this opportunity."

Their glasses clinked.

"And to our engagement...didn't you receive my letter?"

"That's why I came to see you. I needed to talk to you."

"I hope nothing is wrong. I have only received one letter since your return from Arizona."

"I couldn't tell you by letter. I am going steady."

His glass of champagne was poised in midair. "Are you engaged?"

She took a sip of champagne. "His family and my parents have been good friends for a long time. Yes, we are engaged. He is a lieutenant at Wright Field. We will always be good friends."

He ordered two more champagne cocktails.

"Let's dance," she whispered.

They walked to the jukebox, hand in hand. Her light green tailored suit accentuated her graceful figure and the glow of her green eyes. Her beauty was striking and she had class.

"Thanks for the memories. We will always be more than friends," he said. "I haven't heard that tune before. Have you?"

"Try it."

"Won't you tell me when...we will meet again?
Sunday, Monday, or always?..."

"It sounds like Bing Crosby...do you like it?" he asked.

"Yes, and it's wonderful."

"It's wonderful to have you, if only for tonight."

There was a smile upon her lips as she tilted her head back. It was wonderful to have her in his arms again and as they danced, the graceful movement of her body pressed firmly against him.

"Thank you so much," he whispered.

There was a question in her eyes and she smiled. "Sunday, Monday, or always?"

The shadows of twilight were closing in upon them when they started away from the Blue Note, off the main highway, over the back roads and his return. She cuddled close beside him—her touch so warm and caressing. What thrill of excitement was this love they had for each other? A love that was forbidden had been inflamed and intensified by months of pent up passion. A love that made him ache all over. Will I ever see her again? he wondered. He was driving along the country club golf course that was bordered on one side by a large park, just visible in the rising moonlight. She cuddled closer.

"Let's go for a walk in the park," he said as he followed the drive that wound its way through the park. It was just like old times when they had gone driving. Now it seemed like just a short time ago. They reached the crest of a rolling hill that overlooked the lake. There he stopped the car where they could admire the reflection of a rising moon. They remained in a sea of memories and tempting kisses. He was enthralled by her touch, the softness and the smooth satiny feel of her skin, and he loved her firm passionate lips as well as the round firmness of her breasts with nipples that quivered and hardened with his touch. His roaming hands with fingers extended, squeezed about her waist, unfastening the draped around satin blouse, drawing her closer and closer. Soft tantalizing thighs, smooth and silky, surrendered and yielded under pressure. Their whole world throbbed in the darkness that was spinning around and around with caressing lips, possessing and yielding to the ecstasy of life under the starry sky that fell down upon them. This forbidden love was grand and wonderful, and the moments passed swiftly. He had permission to be away from the hospital for the evening. It was past his time for return and he tried to think of some way to prevent her leaving, at least for a little while longer. They left the car and strolled with their arms around each other's waists to a ramada that stood high on the crest of the hill with only the warm breeze to disturb the silence. He was enticed by all her charm, sweetness, and spontaneity in the blissful seclusion. The loving was wonderful.

It was after ten when he started the car and followed the drive out of the park, and then they drove into town where they stopped at a drive-in restaurant. Their order had been taken and they talked about the future. He hoped to be accepted for the engineering course at General Motors. If not, he hadn't firmed up any plans, but now that she was engaged to someone else, he might go to Arizona. It was all so sudden. Until now she had forgotten and there were tears in her eyes as she returned his engagement ring. With the war she didn't know where her marriage would take her. She would go with her husband wherever he had to go, if at all possible. Suddenly, as they were talking about the future, a cab drove up and parked along Pat's side of the car. He would have crawled through the floor of the car, if he could. Miss Barnes and Barton got out of the cab and came up to Pat's side of the car.

"Oh! I thought I recognized one of the nurses," exclaimed Miss Barnes. "The car looks just like Miss Downley's."

Darrell introduced Pat Romane. Then he asked, "How is Miss Downley?"

"She's working at St. Rita's," said Miss Barnes.

Barton introduced her to Pat as Brenda.

"You two sure make a handsome couple," said Brenda.

"Thank you," said Darrell as their order was being served.

"Wouldn't it be wonderful to be young again?" commented

Brenda turning to leave, and to Barton, she added, "Isn't she a beauty? She does resemble Mary Jane Downley."

"Delicious," he said as he swayed toward the cab.

Barton and Brenda were feeling no pain.

It was almost eleven when Darrell and Pat Romane left the drive-in. He had good intentions of returning to the hospital. Pat felt sleepy. It would be a long drive home for Pat at this hour and they decided to stop awhile at the "Rest Haven", a motel that they had passed on their way to town. The room was large with a queen-size bed. They cuddled close to each other with an alluring, fascinating passion, and the loving was more wonderful than before. They slept soundly in each other's arms. Neither one could remember falling asleep. He awoke early and refreshed. His caresses led to more adventurous and passionate lovemaking. It was a night to remember.

Dawn was breaking and it was beginning to rain when they entered the hospital grounds. It was about six o'clock as he drove to the rear entrance of the new building, partly hidden from the watchful eyes of Mr. Beetle. Their farewell exchanges had been made with thanks for the memories and with a hope that somewhere along life's rough and adventurous road they would meet again, as friends or as lovers.

Chapter XXI

LONGER WALKS WITH BETTY

The next morning Darrell was awakened by the voice of Pap Henry. He had dozed off for about twenty minutes. It was strange to hear Pap's voice on a Saturday morning. Maw and Pap had changed their day off, which was unusual. It was almost seven, and it was raining. Pap had a good voice, very strong, and he continued to sing as he adjusted the windows:

"...Singing in the rain...Oh what a
glorious feeling....just singing in the rain..."

Frequently Pap would sing in the mornings as he closed the windows or adjusted them in the early morning hours. And this morning his voice was exceptionally good.

Oh! What a glorious feeling! This feeling of love was grand, exciting, and exhilarating. It was fun while it lasted. What memories! That's life! And it was wonderful to be alive.

His thoughts were interrupted by Maw who was taking the pulses. She looked at him questionably. "Your pulse is higher than normal. I need to take your temperature too."

The temperatures were taken every other day, not on Saturday or Sunday, and he wondered why. He felt fine and he was hungry.

"I was dreaming."

"I told you that you shouldn't read those racy, sexy novels. It's not good for a patient like you; too exciting." Maw returned for his temperature reading. "Your temperature is normal. That's good."

"I was thinking about what I'll do when I'm released. I had some disappointing news, but I feel relieved and much better now."

"Don't think about it."

"Oh! I won't. I feel fine!"

At breakfast he had a double serving of eggs. Pap was accommodating occasionally, and he had requested second servings. There was no indication that Maw or Pap had noticed his late return last night, or rather early this morning. Only Barton knew his secret and Barton had come in late, but much earlier than Darrell. Barton told him that Miss Barnes had wanted to warn him that she wouldn't be on duty today, but it had slipped her mind. When he asked about Pat, Darrell told him that their engagement was broken. During the morning rest hour he lay quietly to rest and soon fell asleep with dreams of last night. He also slept through the afternoon rest hour. Later in the day he wrote a letter to Pat thanking her for the wonderful, unforgettable evening, a night to remember, and that she had given to his life a very special touch which meant so much. He hoped that she would keep in touch.

Sometimes Darrell took long walks alone in the afternoon to the golf course where it was delightful to feel the soft, even grass on the fairways. Occasionally he would walk through the park to the crest of the high rolling hill and the ramada overlooking the lake where he could sit down to rest. There his thoughts wandered and he was alone with the memories of a night that once was so full of happiness. The walks helped him to regain strength, both physically and mentally, for now he had to come down to earth and make life anew. Life was there for the living while it could be enjoyed. What was done could not be undone. An old, grade school teacher had told him, "Don't cry over spilled milk." Darrell continued to receive pneumos, but only 75 to 100 cc's of air as his lung continued to expand, forcing its way out with the added exercise.

The weekly radio broadcasts continued with Darrell as the announcer. Betty Gordon helped to change records. Except for the records that his sister had given him, there were no new records. In order to develop more interest and to get more participation, one act plays were dramatized and poems were submitted and read. Even Miss Bellhaven took more of an interest and enjoyed the broadcasts. She knew several of the members of the women's club and he persuaded her to contact them for a contribution for some newer records. It was only after the weekly broadcast that the patients were permitted out after dusk and that was only for the return of the women to the old building. As the days grew longer and the weather became warmer, some of the patients began to stay out later in the evenings. Mr. Beetle detected their late return and a curfew hour was established. Occasionally, Weasel-face could be seen snooping around the darkened corners of the ivy walls.

As the days became warmer and he was raised in class, he began to take longer walks with Betty Gordon through the park and its adjoining dense wooded area. The outdoor exercise was wonderful. Just being able to be out of bed meant so very much: the feel of the breeze upon their faces; the grass beneath their feet; and the trees above with the leaves fluttering in the breeze. The walks were carefree and happy, filled with a desire of love as they wandered hand in hand along the trails where the sun filtered through the leaves. The only noise that was heard was the rustling of the leaves, the chirps and twittering calls of the birds, the chirps of the crickets and grasshoppers, and their own laughter. It was a waiting game and they enjoyed each other's company as they shared their hospital experiences.

About the middle of June, Bill Read visited Darrell. He had been to the clinic for pneumothorax treatment and X-rays.

"I'm leaving in a week for Phoenix, Arizona. Do you want to come along?"

"I wish I could."

"Doc gave me the X-ray which I got this morning to take along and he also gave me the name of a good doctor who he knows in Phoenix. He said he has a clinic in a professional building in Phoenix. It'll cost me five bucks a shot for pneumos and I need pneumos every ten days. They didn't cost me anything here, but I can't spend another hay fever season here and I'll need X-rays every six months. I don't believe Arizona has any assistance program like we have in Ohio and I won't be eligible to receive any assistance since I'm not able to qualify as a legal resident. Doc warned me that I couldn't let any of my treatments lapse; the next two years will be critical. I'll need pneumos every ten days for the next three years or more."

"How are you going?"

Read laughed. "I'm gonna hitchhike. If I get stranded, I'll take a bus."

"Won't that be too much for you?"

"I'm working six hours a day now and next month Doc says that I should be able to work eight. That's why I waited until now to go west. Wait until you get out. It's really rough when one can work only four hours a day...and that strange look of fear you will see when you tell them that you have had TB. What do you plan to do when you're released?"

"I'll try again for that engineering training program."

"Wouldn't you have to work full time?"

"If I can't qualify, I may go west too."

"I'll write and let you know how I'm doing. Are you still getting pneumos?"

"Yes, but I'm losing my air space. I've got one lung to go. Doc says he'll give me a phrenic when my lung comes out. I hope that I don't get fluid again. Will your Dad be going to Arizona too?"

"He plans to come out later, after I see what the job situation is. He prefers Colorado where my aunt lives, but we believe that Arizona will be better for us."

Bill Reed had spent more than two and a half years in the sanatorium. He was well liked by all who knew him and he seemed to know everyone in the new building. He was invited to stay for lunch and left shortly thereafter with best wishes from all, including Maw and Pap Henry. For them it was a pleasure to see any of the old graduates, as they were called, who were doing well. For most it had been a long, long time before they had been declared arrested or free from infection and safe to be out among their friends and the public.

Darrell was now in class ten and Betty Gordon was in class twelve. She would be released within another two months and as their walks became longer, she talked of her life that had once been filled with happiness. And now that her engagement had been broken, she didn't plan to get involved again, not for some time—just friends, but no ties. Darrell told her of his broken engagement and that after fourteen months under the present circumstances, he couldn't blame Pat, for this was no life to offer. Then one day on a long, long walk when they sat down to rest and relax, his lips searched for hers and met them with heated passion. Their lips met again playfully, more passionately in soft caresses. As they struggled in their playful game, their hearts beat faster and faster, and her breasts heaved under pressure. Under the spell, his senses were aflamed with the loveliness of her body as he kissed her lips, her ears, her throat, and all the alluring beauty of her breasts. A violent throbbing welled-up within to the movements of her hips, her thighs, and her legs. They clung to each other with tremulous lips in the smooth surging rhythm of vibrant passion, rolling, swelling, surging with all the life possessed in grasping, seizing moments. Then all was quiet and they lay in each other's arms, lip to lip in long tender kisses where love was wonderful with the never ending desire for all the charm and unknown delights that were discovered.

The walk back that day was longer still, like ten miles. But life was wonderful and the days drifted. Days when they met were shortened by the love they had for each other. A love where each surrender was more thrilling and yet they knew it could not be, it should not be, for what chance had this life and love of theirs for the future? But life was made to be lived and to be enjoyed, they told each other, and these precious, stolen moments were not claimed and should not be wasted, but enjoyed to the fullest.

Toward the last of June when he was being fluoroscoped, Doctor Sheridan said, "You have fluid again—not very much, not enough to draw off. I won't give you any air today, maybe next week. Continue with your exercise."

He was now in class eleven and with the coming of July, another round of sputum checks was taken.

July, with its hot and humid days, carried with it the saddened spirits of the fellows at the new building. However there were more fellows who had entered with only a slight infection; fellows who had failed to pass their army physical. They were the more fortunate ones, whose illness had been discovered before it had advanced. They showed fast improvement with the proper food and rest and if necessary, pneumothorax treatment. They were an added encouragement to the doctors and nurses. Not so for the old lungers who were almost like fixtures, waiting with little or no change and watching as the fortunate ones pass them by, left with the memories of their youth that had once meant health; health that was lost or stolen away. Time meant little to them. What really mattered was the hope that someday they would regain their health and it was a real pleasure to take long walks in clean fresh air.

These were the fellows who took their places among the old lungers that still remained on the west side where a gloomy atmosphere hung as a result of a positive sputum check.

Miss Bellhaven, who supervised the weekly broadcasts, had informed Darrell that he could buy some records at the "Music Box" and charge them to the women's club. Higgins offered to take him to town the next afternoon that his wife visited him. That day, Skinner ate very little. The positive report was disheartening.

"Paul, why don't you eat your food?" asked Maw. "You don't eat enough to keep a bird alive."

"I won't get well anyway," retorted Skinner.

"Oh, you might!" she taunted.

With his eyes veiled in tears, Skinner had pleaded with Doctor Sheridan for permission to remain at the new building, but that was impossible. Maw had insisted that it was difficult for him to obtain the proper rest. With the newer group of fellows there was more activity. They had more visitors and often left the sanatorium in the afternoon and evening for a drive into town or around the countryside. Skinner couldn't stay a day longer. After the noon meal with his head hung down in silence, Skinner began the long, long road that became lonelier each time it had to be retraced. Two of the fellows on the east side were positive and they too had to take the long, long trip.

Darrell walked with Skinner to the elevator of the old sanatorium. Of the five on the sunporch when he had entered, only two had not had to make the return trip. Bunnigan had obtained an early release when he was caught out after hours with Dorothy Marline and Darrell was now in class eleven. The odds weren't good. Darrell felt deeply grieved, for he and Skinner had traveled through the classes together. The sunporch experiences could not be easily forgotten. Randall had been so serious and read his Bible fervently before he had been wheeled out toes up. Towers worried but joked and laughed, which seemed to help. Skinner has what it takes. He'll make it, Darrell thought as he waited for the elevator door to close. He then decided to go to the library and he entered the rear entrance.

At the library he met Patricia Brentwood. She was now in class seven and had planned to come to the next broadcast. He asked if she had a favorite song that she would like to have played.

"Yes, play Stardust for me."

"It isn't available in our record collection, but when I go to town, I'll buy it. We have received a donation from the women's club. Miss Bellhaven was helpful in arranging it for us."

They talked about Skinner and she asked about his girl. He sounded very serious as he talked of their broken engagement and their night out.

"Don't take it so serious," she said with a laugh. "You"ll come out of it alive. I had a broken marriage and the world didn't come to an end."

Patricia Brentwood was looking much better after her rib surgery and talked about outdoor exercise. She knew what it was like to have a relapse as had happened to Skinner. The percent of breakdowns was as great for women as for men. The facilities were hot and crowded, and there was a shortage of qualified doctors and nurses. Doctor Schmidt and family had returned to India. Doctor Sheridan was alone. The local hospital staff doctors helped in an emergency and in surgery.

When Darrell returned to the west side, Higgins said, "This place gives me the creeps."

"Yeah, with every check somebody gets knocked off," added Millford.

"It's really hot and crowded at the old building. When are you going to be released, Higgins?" asked Darrell.

Higgins smiled from ear to ear. "Next week."

"Hell, Doc wanted to release him two months ago," bantered Millford, "but Higgins is afraid of his shadow. As long as his insurance is paying, he'll stay."

"When I go home," retorted Higgins, "I want to be able to work."

"As soon as I get my final check," said Millford, "I'm getting the hell out of here."

"Doc told me that I could work four hour a day and what kind of a damn job would I do for four hours a day? My old boss would laugh at me."

"I'll find something to do," said Millford. "It's getting so a guy can't even turn around here anymore. Old Weasel-face stopped me yesterday when I was walking toward the Alpine and wanted to know where I was going."

"This place isn't the same anymore with so many of the old gang missing," commented Barton.

"How's Blake doing?" asked Darrell.

"He went negative after his second stage of ribs," replied Barton.

"What about Towers?"

"He's negative...ought to be raised in class in another month."

"I'll have to stop and visit the old gang or at least the fellows on the surgery ward. I suppose Transfusion is still roaming the halls."

"He tried to commit suicide several days ago, but the nurse discovered it in time. He had slashed his wrist with a razor," concluded Barton.

The following afternoon, when rest hour was over, Darrell went to town with Higgins and his wife. They stopped at the "Music Box" where he selected four records:

Stay As Sweet As You Are

In The Mood
Stardust, and
Blueberry Hill.

On their return, they stopped at St. Rita's Hospital to see Mary Jane Downley. She was in surgery. He left a note thanking her for the special care and help that she had given him and he hoped to see her on his next visit.

"Lucky in cards! Unlucky in love!" exclaimed Higgins.

"I'll try again," said Darrell. "She is a very special nurse; someone I'll never forget."

"Miss Barnes is a friend of hers. She can get in touch with her," said Higgins.

"Thanks, I'll see what develops."

Darrell and Higgins returned to the new building in time for the five o'clock supper. Later that evening a cab stopped at the nurses' building and followed the circular drive around to the men's building. Barton had dressed hurriedly and rushed to the cab where Miss Barnes waited. He was excited by the thrill of getting away as he leaned back to relax. Then out from a darkened corner, a flashlight beamed.

"Don't stop for him," commanded Barton as he sank to the floor behind the driver. But Beetle ran into the path of the cab, waving his flashlight wildly. Barton's heart beat rapidly as the brakes were applied. "You damn fool!" shouted Barton, "I told you not to stop."

It was too late. The light flashed in his eyes and he was caught like a mouse in a trap as Beetle glared from Barton to Miss Barnes.

"Get out!" he shouted.

"Get away from my cab," she yelled, "or I'll flatten you!"

"You're fired!" shouted Beetle.

"You have a nerve. You can't fire me. I don't work for you. I have a right to go to town and besides, I wouldn't work for you!"

"As for you,"' he continued, glaring at Barton with his beady eyes, "pack your clothes and get out."

"He has my permission to share this cab. Get away from my cab," shouted Miss Barnes.

The driver of the cab sat fidgety, glancing from one to the other.

"You damn idiot! Drive on, if you want to get paid," she commanded.

The motor roared and with a lunge the cab spurted ahead, leaving Mr. Beetle waving his flashlight.

Barton didn't return until the afternoon of the following day and after checking with Doctor Sheridan for a final examination, X-ray and blood test, he stopped for his luggage.

"Beetle got us last night," said Barton in a very quiet voice to Darrell. "I told that cab driver not to stop, but he did. He must have been a friend of Beetle's. You and Betty had better watch out."

"We are. We try to keep respectable hours," said Darrell with a wink. "What about Brenda?"

"Doc told her that he wouldn't fire her, that he needs her, and that since I'm leaving, it may appease Beetle. I could have stayed if I wanted, but I only had five weeks remaining before my scheduled release. Brenda may go to work at St. Rita's."

Chapter XXII

AN ESCAPE AND GOING HOME PARTY AT THE ALPINE

When Darrell went to the clinic that week, Miss Barnes was working with Doctor Sheridan. He was teaching her the proper procedures for pneumothorax treatment in the event of an emergency. Darrell's lung was of particular interest since his diaphragm had creeped up along his pleural wall, and extreme care was necessary to insert the needle at the proper place and angle to reach the small pocket of fluid. His side was aspirated. The fluid that was drawn off was purulent. It was a small amount, about 75 cc's, and his side was irrigated with the Azoclorarnid solution and about 100 cc's of air was induced. He told Doctor Sheridan that even though his temperature had risen to 100.2, his appetite was good and he managed to eat fairly well. As instructed, he waited in the adjoining room until he was fluoroscoped to see how much air space he had. There was no opportunity to talk with Miss Barnes about the recent escapade or Miss Downley, as the number of patients awaiting pneumos was unusually large.

In his walk away from the clinic toward the second floor

surgery ward and sunporch, he stopped at the fourth cubbyhole. There, enclosed by side boards, lay a skeleton framework of skin and bones too feeble to climb out. His drawn and sunken eyelids opened, uncovering a pair of sunken beady eyes.

"How are you, Darrell?" came a weak, almost silent voice through his drawn lips and sunken mouth.

"Fine, except I've got a recurrence of fluid and empyema. I'm in class eleven. I should be released in about three months."

"I'm waiting for my release too," said Transfusion, "toes up!" And he managed to add a chuckle, as was his habit.

"Don't give up the ship. Hang in there. Medical research is searching for that magical drug."

"This ship is already sinking with this ill-fated fortune," said Transfusion, then chuckled: "I've already sent up the flares."

"Maybe they'll see the light," said Darrell turning toward the open doorway.

What a pitiful sight, Darrell thought as he walked away. With all the resistance that he once had, Transfusion, who had gone until he couldn't go anymore, certainly wasn't going to beat this plague. Visible on his wrist was the scar of his attempted suicide. Rounding the corridor, Darrell entered the sunporch. Skinner had Darrell's old bed in the corner by the windows where he had spent almost a year. From the windows he could see the nurses' building to the east and the men's building to the west. Towers had Randall's bed. The other three beds were occupied by three other unfortunate victims, all in their twenties.

"How's life along 'Commodilly Row'?"

Towers laughed. "We don't have any commodes on the sunporch anymore."

"Where's Marrow?"

"About six feet under!" exclaimed Skinner.

"He took his ribs with him," added Towers. "Spit a hemorrhage across the room about two weeks ago. It wouldn't stop."

"What about Blande? Was he transferred to a private room?"

"Heart stopped!" replied Skinner. "He had no sense of humor as you well know. He couldn't take it. He had high blood pressure, poor circulation and a weak heart."

Darrell laughed. "It takes a mighty strong constitution, a great heart with a lot of courage, and determination to beat this plague. It takes even more to stay well. A good sense of humor helps."

"You said it. I made a cure, or an apparent cure, five years ago, and I was up to class eleven when I had to return for thoracoplasty," said Towers.

"What class are you in?"

"I was raised to class three yesterday."

"How about you, Paul?"

"I had a negative check. One more and I'll be on my way up again. I couldn't believe that positive check."

Towers chuckled, "Those little tubercle bacilli don't lie."

"And they don't lie idle either," said Darrell, turning to leave with farewells to Towers, Skinner and the three new unfortunate victims who enjoyed their exchange of comments.

Walking down the corridor, Darrell hesitated as he was about to pass the first private room on the right. A gaunt, sallow-faced fellow lay there with his eyes closed; his cheekbones protruded under his drawn, pale skin. He was almost too weak to take thoracoplasty. Time was running out as he lay there and wasted away. Youth was losing another bout unless some miraculous drug came along soon.

When he entered the room, Robbins opened his eyes.

"Hello, Robbins," said Darrell in a whispering voice.

"Good to see you. Read said you might go to Arizona."

"I don't intend to go unless I'm unable to land that job with GM."

"If you do, be sure that you're able or well enough to make the trip. Don't do as I did and ride straight through."

"Do you have any requests for the broadcast tonight?"

"Would you read two or three of the verses from The Rubaiyat of Omar Khayyam? I have the book from the library which I was about to return."

"Sure, and I'll return it to the librarian for you."

"And play a couple of Spike Jones recordings: Pass the Biscuits, Mirandi and Cocktails For Two. I almost fell out of bed when you first played them. I thought I'd die laughing. They are really crazy, lively tunes."

That Friday evening at the broadcast, Darrell read three verses from The Rubaiyat of Omar Khayyam.

"Oh, my Beloved, fill the cup that clears
today of past regrets and future fears—
Tomorrow? Why, Tomorrow I may be
myself with yesterday's seven thousand years.

Myself when young did eagerly frequent
doctor and saint, and heard great argument
about it and about: but evermore
came out by the same door as in I went.

Come, fill the cup, and in the fire of spring
the winter garment of repentance fling;
the bird of time has but a little way
to fly-and lo! The bird is on the wing."

It was a happy evening at the broadcast. Several of the women were going home next week, including Betty Gordon and Phyliss Carlyle. They were singing and having a grand time. Higgins and Millford were also going home Sunday and Milford had arranged a going home party at the Alpine for Friday night. They didn't have much to loose if they were caught out after nine. Patricia Brentwood was helping to select and change records, and he played Stardust for her:

"...Sometimes I wonder why I spend
each lonely night dreaming of a song...
The melody haunts my reverie and
I am once again with you..."

In return she selected an old record for him and she announced it as, I'll String Along With You:

"...I'm looking for an angel,
but angels are so few...
So just until the day that one comes along,
I'll string along with you..."

The records requested by Robbins were played and by special request he played Stay As Sweet As You Are for the nurses. The station signed off at eight o'clock, as usual. He showed Patricia Brentwood around the west side before he escorted her back to the old building and told her about the gang who were going to slip out later for the going home party. She had already heard about it and decided that the walk would be too much now. Miss Bellhaven made sure that those who had attended, returned to their respective rooms before nine.

Shortly after nine, Milford, Higgins and Darrell made their way through the darkness, Indian style, along the trail that led far around to the east of the sanatorium and then north along the fence to the rear of Doctor Sheridan's house. Occasionally Millford, who was leading the way, turned as he walked, calling to the fellows to step it up. The trail was scarcely visible and Higgins, who was following close behind Millford, stopped abruptly.

"Come on, I know t-h-," Millford's voice trailed sway.

Higgins and Darrell stared down at Millford who picked himself up from where he had rolled, fifteen feet from the top of the ravine.

"Are you all right?" asked Darrell.

Higgins was laughing his head off. "That's the same place where he fell before. You'd think he would wise up."

Millford brushed off the dust and dirt and shook himself.

Higgins waved his left arm and yelled, "Come on, I know the way."

After much laughter, slipping and sliding, they scampered up the other side.

"That's no climb for a blind man," said Darrell.

Millford was puffing on one lung. "That's no climb for an ole lunger like me."

"Nor for a young ole lunger. It's rough with only one lung working!" exclaimed Darrell.

"My heart is pounding," added Higgins, "and I've got a pain in my prostate."

"That's a new wrinkle," said Darrell with a laugh. "Maybe you better not go home. You haven't been taking your exercise."

Darrell had not gone for any long walks for the past several days because of the reoccurrence of his fluid. However his temperature had dropped back to normal and he wanted to go to the going home party. Betty Gordon was leaving soon and she was to meet him there.

"Let's go! The women will be waiting," said Millford, leading the way over the pathway that was barely visible in the tall grass.

"Are there any snakes in here?" asked Higgins.

"No, this is too close to the old sanatorium for snakes. They won't be out at night," said Darrell in a joking manner, as if the sanatorium could protect them from snakes of any kind.

Shortly after ten they entered the nightclub. Smoke hung around the dim lights like layers of screens from the low ceiling. A row of fellows and several gals who lined the bar stools stared at them as if they were convicts, then returned to their drinks. The odor of beer and whiskey was heavy and the music of the nickelodeon was heard above the din of laughter. Four couples were dancing as the fellows proceeded toward the table where four women sat along the wall next to the dance floor. The waitress stood by and eyed them curiously as they pushed two tables together.

"You're new here, aren't you?" queried Millford impressively. She ignored his question and asked to see his draft card. "I'll be damn," he said, turning to the fellows, "I'm thirty-four and she doesn't think that I'm twenty-one."

"Let's see your draft card."

"How do you like that? I left it at the club in my wallet."

"I can't serve you."

"But I'm thirty-four. Here take a look at my teeth!"
Millford pulled out his upper plate and waved them in mid-air.

The bartender laughed. "I know him."

The laughs were on Millford. He was burning, but it was comical and the laughter around the table rang loud. After the round of beers was ordered, Millford discovered that he had lost his girl's ring and Higgins related how he had disappeared before him and rolled down the ravine.

After several rounds of beer, everyone was in a happy, relaxed mood. It was wonderful after a long, long time to be able to be going home, and tonight, to be away from the sanatorium. Just being somewhere that when they shouldn't be added to their celebration and gaiety. For the six who were leaving, the average time spent in the sanatorium was more than two and one-half years. Darrell felt like one of them. It was a special occasion and for each it meant a complete break with the past, a challenge to be out on their own, to earn a living, and most important of all, to live a healthy life. A real test confronted them, which required the help of relatives and friends. It meant a proper diet, regular hours for rest, and peace of mind.

Phyliss Carlyle, a slender brunette who was dancing with Millford to the beat of "Pistol Packing Mama," had a puzzled look on her face as Higgins, who was seated at the table with Margie, a redhead in her early thirties, and Lucille, a light complexioned girl with coal black hair, were laughing at Millford's pajamas that hung an inch below his trousers. What a sight it was! Darrell, who was dancing with Betty Gordon, looked, but couldn't tell if his pajamas were noticeable too.

A big burly fellow asked Lucille for a dance. They danced to several tunes. He wanted to take her home. Everything was fine until she told him that she was in the sanatorium and had to return. She was attractive, in her twenties.

"I thought that I had a ride," said Lucille, "but he looked as if I had shot him out of the saddle. Why, he dropped me like a hot potato when I told him that I had to return to the sanatorium," she said and laughed as her blue eyes glistened.

Darrell began to sing and they all joined in:

"...Lay that pistol down Babe,
lay that pistol down.
Pistol Packing Mama,
lay that pistol down..."

They left the Alpine after several more dances and another round of beers. A moon was breaking out between a cloudy sky that partially hid the stars from view. The night air was clean and fresh with the summer breeze that had a strange, sweet fragrant smell, after the stale air of the nightclub and the medicinal air of the sanatorium. Millford and Phyliss, arm in arm, led the way down the narrow trail singing:

"Show me the way to go home.
I'm tired and I wanna go to bed.

Had a little drink about an hour ago,
and it went right to my head..."

Margie, Lucille and Higgins followed them. They all joined in the singing as Betty and Darrell brought up the rear, hand in hand, thighs and hips brushing. When they reached the ravine, they all paused. Out of the stilled darkness there came a beaming, flashing light and the shrill blast of a whistle with the rumbling wheels of the train.

"Doesn't the fire look wonderful?" asked Betty.

"The flames are even coming out of its smokestack."

They waited on top until the train passed while the others climbed down the side of the ravine. Like two lovers lost in a blanket of darkness and sweet caresses, they clung to each other in long tender kisses, for they knew that this was to be their farewell and they lingered there a while longer. After days and weeks of sharing the sad experiences of the sanatorium, it was so sudden, this departure that they knew was inevitable and had to be. For her, this release from the sanatorium meant a new life and they had agreed to go their separate ways.

Then, slipping and sliding, they reached the bottom of the ravine. Suddenly, she grabbed his arm tightly. "Look Joe! A couple of fellows are coming across the tracks."

As he peered at the shadowy figures, his muscles tensed. His heart was pounding fast as they drew nearer. "That's Millford and Phyliss."

"Oh, you scared us!" said Betty as they approached.

"We thought you two lovers were lost," said Phyliss. "Margie, Lucille and Higgins are waiting on top."

The climb was steep and the loose gravel was slippery. At the top they stopped to catch their breath, for at best, they each had one lung working. Slowly they followed the pathway, singing in individual refrain as they walked along:

"Row, row, row your boat,
gently down the stream...
merrily, merrily, merrily, merrily,
life is but a dream..."

When the sanatorium appeared in the light of the moon, their voices became softer, then silent. They proceeded ever so softly until they embraced with parting farewells; the beginning of a grand and glorious freedom; a life to live again.

Chapter XXIII

A NIGHT OUT WITH PATRICIA BRENTWOOD

Shortly after midnight the women entered the rear door of the sanatorium that had been purposely left unlocked. The fellows continued along the shadows of the wooded area that bordered the circular drive to the rear entrance of the new building. Only a faint light glowed from Mr. Beetle's house that was located just beyond a small pond extending along the west side of the new building. They tiptoed into the washroom and undressed to their pajamas. Millford was hungry and decided to raid the kitchen. They hadn't raided the kitchen since Bunnigan had left, when according to Barton, Miss Barnes had said that Maw was getting suspicious and warned them that she couldn't cover for them any longer, and that Maw thought that Bunnigan was responsible. After Millford opened the dutch door, Darrell and Higgins joined him in the kitchen where the three ate a dozen eggs, two thick slices of ham, a whole apple pie and a quart of ice cream between them. Millford and Higgins said that they would take the blame if Maw missed the ice cream.

The next day Miss Barnes worked for Maw and Pap. Darrell had become more acquainted. She said that she had seen Barton last week. He had returned to his plumbing business, working part-time, and he was doing well. When Darrell asked about Miss Downley, she said that she was working full time, doing well, not a trace of any infection, and that she was going steady with one of the interns at St. Rita's Hospital. With a wink she said that it shouldn't prevent him from seeing her.

He slept soundly through the two-hour rest period from one to three, a much needed relaxing rest before he would meet Patricia Brentwood for a short walk. Two blocks away from the sanatorium grounds they met and walked arm in arm. She was attractive in her street clothes. With her shapely figure, her rib surgery wasn't evident. They were excited as he talked about the going home party last night. Phyliss and Betty had already left earlier that afternoon. Their walk led to the park where they rested at the ramada overlooking the lake. They wanted to walk further, but her exercise time was limited. There were several small rowboats on the lake and only a few Saturday afternoon visitors as they lingered there enjoying the picturesque view and each other's company.

Sunday afternoon, after rest hour, Higgins and Millford left for home. Higgins was grinning from ear to ear, showing a mouthful of white, even teeth, as he waved good-bye to the fellows. They lined the walk at the rear entrance, clad in colorful pajamas. Mrs. Higgins, a tall, slender, cheerful woman, shook hands with Darrell and exchanged best wishes. It was a joyous occasion. A released patient seldom made a return visit except for an X-ray or treatments. Millford, who didn't have a family, rode to town with Higgins and his wife. He had a part-time job as a hotel clerk and planned to get a room at a small hotel near work. Both had to readjust to a new routine and work after three years of bed rest in the sanatorium. These would be trying times for both, but much more difficult for Millford who didn't have a steady, regular home life, and who always had to have entertainment or some other activity going to create interest or excitement and release nervous energy.

Darrell was the last of the old lungers who remained on the west side. Two young fellows, about Darrell's age, were transferred to the west side from the old building. They were avid poker players, and for some of the games, the limit was raised from ten cents to twenty-five cents. They played every chance they had throughout the day. Occasionally, Darrell would play in the evenings. He had a lucky streak and was about seventy dollars ahead. They were a carefree happy group, unlike the old lungers who seemed afraid or constrained to the exercise within their classification. Sundays were reserved for visitors and a drive into town or the countryside. Darrell had few visitors. Occasionally, he was invited to go along for a drive when someone was needed to complete a foursome. They would stop at the Alpine, the Blue Note or some other clubs in town for an afternoon round of refreshments and dancing to the nickelodeon. It was great fun and the development of good friendships. He had written home to advise them of the Sunday afternoon activities and to coordinate visits of relatives and friends. When Darrell had no visitors on Sunday afternoons, he took long walks alone in the park, along the lake, and deeper into the wooded area. He was alone with his thoughts born of a life that he had lost—lost youth and a beautiful, lovely girl. These were joyful thoughts, in a way, for love had been grand and it was better to have loved than never to have loved at all.

Sometimes during the week when he met Patricia Brentwood, they would walk along some of the trails that he had discovered. It was quiet and peaceful with only the breeze in the tip-top of oak and hickory trees, the mating call of the birds and the "poom-poom-poom" chatter of the squirrels to disturb the stillness. They talked quietly of the little things that they enjoyed and it was wonderful to be together and to become more acquainted. There was a different, glorious feeling of love, a common bond brought about by a quiet understanding of two persons thrown together by a destiny of ill-fated fortune.

August arrived. Joe was somewhat concerned about the recurrence of empyema that hadn't cleared and the fact that his lung was forcing its way out against his pleural wall as it had done last August. The following week about 50 cc's of purulent fluid were drawn off and his pleural cavity was irrigated with Azocloramid solution. He was thankful that this medication was helping his body to contain the infection.

"We'll let your lung come out," said Doctor Sheridan, "and then we'll give you a phrenic. I believe that will check your fluid."

He paused as he studied the expressed disappointment on Darrell's face. Darrell thought that his lung had not healed sufficiently, and he didn't like what he had heard and seen. The greenish-yellow fluid was sickening and his temperature had risen again to more then 100. However his body had developed its own way to fight off the infection, given time, proper rest, and a good diet. The thoughts of others, like Bunnigan who had made it with a phrenic alone after his lung had come out, were comforting. Doctor Sheridan continued in a confident and heartening tone of voice. "You've done well. Continue to take your exercise as you have been doing. What class are you in?"

"Eleven. I enjoy the walking exercise."

"We'll raise you to class twelve. You should take about three hours of walking exercise each day, moderate speed."

"How long will I have to remain in class twelve?"

Doctor Sheridan's eyes opened wide with a rather questioning look. Finally he replied, "Three months, but don't get impatient. You're infection was moderately advanced. Three more months now will give you time to build up your strength so that you will be better prepared for a real adjustment when you are released. The change in hours and work when you are on your own with all the other temptations will be difficult to cope with. There are many here who don't take the proper amount of rest or exercise. They haven't learned to relax and quit worrying. As I mentioned some time ago, these are the ones that make up the majority of the fifty percent who have a relapse within the first two years. We don't want that to happen to you. I've received many good comments on the weekly broadcast from the patients," continued Doctor Sheridan, changing the subject. "They like the records and the poems."

"Most of the recordings are in answer to requests that we received and some have been donated by the women's club. May I have your permission to go to town for some other records?"

"Yes, and I have an advance article on some research that is being done by Doctor Waksman who has isolated streptomycin, for you to read. It will be encouraging to the patients to hear what is being done by medical research. The drug is low toxicity and has been found to be effective in experimental animals against tubercle bacilli. Many rumors about streptomycin are being circulated. Previous drugs have been disappointing, but we believe that this will be effective. However, it will be limited and expensive. It will also be some time before it is fully tested and available for use by physicians. If we are successful, it will mean that long months or years of bed rest and some pneumothorax treatment will not be necessary. That doesn't mean that bed rest and proper diet won't be required. The public won't have to fear the disease as we now know it."

"That's good news. Some of the released patients tell about the difficult times they have to find work and the fear others have when they learn that they have had TB."

"Control, we believe, is in sight. We will eventually find a drug that is non-toxic. There will continue to be a stigma attached to it that will take time to overcome; time to educate the public about environmental health and the air we breathe."

Doctor Sheridan paused, then continued, "The local chapter of the National Tuberculosis Association has heard about the weekly broadcast and wants to extend the power transmitting capability. The broadcast signal can only be picked up in the nearby vicinity, a few blocks from the sanatorium. They have a few records that have been donated by some of the members, which they are sending out to me and I'll give them to you or send them over. We are also checking into the possibility of increasing the signal."

Leaving the office, his footsteps retraced the same old corridors through which he had shuffled on his way to the bathroom. Passing the cubbyholes on his left, he saw strange pale faces. He paused at the fourth cubbyhole. Transfusion was not there. He had obtained his release "toes up!" He had gone until he could go no more. There was no effective medicine and his body, once strong and efficient, could withstand no more. Farewell, old friend, he thought.

On the sunporch, Towers, who was in class five, was waiting to be transferred to the new building again as soon as a bed became available. Skinner still had Darrell's old bed in the corner. He was as spunky as always and talked about starting up in class again after more than four years. Blake had been moved into the middle bed following his thoracoplasty. All three were in a relatively good mood considering the time that each had spent there. When Darrell left the sunporch, he walked slowly toward the first private room. Robbins was too weak to move about or to get out of bed. The drug that Doctor Sheridan had talked about wouldn't be available soon enough. He was reading some of the poems of Henry W. Longfellow. Darrell entered and Robbins asked him to read two verses from The Goblet of Life at the weekly broadcast, and also to play the record, I'm Going Back To Where I Come From. The color of Robbins' skin was even more sallow than before. It was an effort for him to speak and he talked in a whisper and gave a weak, feeble laugh when Darrell told him how Millford had fallen down the ravine on the way to the going home party at the Alpine. Maw had convinced him not to have thoracoplasty, but he was full of praise for Maw Henry.

That Friday evening Darrell announced the broadcast as emanating from the beautiful shores of "Moonlight Bay" alongside an old ivy-walled sanatorium. The first song selected by Patricia Brentwood was On Moonlight Bay:

"...You have stolen my heart,
now don't go away,
as we sing love's old sweet song
on Moonlight Bay..."

There was much laughing and joking about going away from the sanatorium by those attending the broadcast. Darrell read the encouraging article about streptomycin that Doctor Sheridan had given him. And there was more laughter when he announced Robbins' request, I'm Going Back To Where I Come From. A silent mood prevailed as he read three verses from The Goblet of Life:

"Then in life's goblet freely press,
the leaves that give it bitterness,
nor prize the colored waters less,
for in thy darkness and distress,
new light and strength they give!

And he who has not learned to know
how false its sparkling bubbles show,
how bitter are the drops of woe,
with which its brim may overflow,
he has not learned to live.

I pledge you in this cup of grief,
where floats the fennel's bitter leaf.
The battle of our life is brief,
the alarm, the struggle, the relief,
then sleep we side by side."

Then to enliven the listeners he changed the tempo with In The Mood and Chattanooga Choo Choo, followed by requests from the spectators, which included:

You Are My Sunshine,
Paper Doll,
Apple Blossom Time, and
Don't Get Around Much Anymore

And he played a special song, Blueberry Hill, for Patricia Brentwood that reminded him of their walk by the hill overlooking the lake. After the broadcast they chatted leisurely as they awaited the return of one of several of the umbrellas that was being used to escort the women back to the old building, for it had begun to rain. When he mentioned that he had received permission to go to town for some records, she suggested that they go together some Saturday afternoon. A Saturday would be best for her and she planned to get permission to visit home. He said that it would be great and that they would finalize the time when they met for their walk tomorrow afternoon if the weather cleared. It was nearing nine o'clock when they started out into the drizzling rain, and she snuggled close under the umbrella. The misty drizzle seemed to hang in gleaning beams from the glowing light of the windows and they walked slowly toward the sheltered passageway with an arm around each other's waist. They lingered in the sheltered passageway by the elevator. Their goodnight kisses were exciting. Approaching footsteps could be heard. The elevator door closed and she disappeared as the small glass window of the door passed beyond the upper ledge. Miss Bellhaven and Mrs. Kenny entered hurriedly. He greeted them and proceeded out into the drizzling rain under the protection of the umbrella. He walked along with a burning, throbbing numbness. The light of a flashlight beamed on the old wooden bridge that crossed a narrow neck of the small lake and he hurried his steps. It was after nine o'clock. Who would care to be out on a night like this? He could barely make out the slim, sneaking figure of Mr. Beetle as he passed through the reflected light from the windows.

Late that Friday evening, Robbins died. There was no one there, but on the nightstand beside his bed was a note of thanks to Darrell.

Saturday the weather was still rainy and he spent the afternoon playing bridge with the fellows. They met Monday afternoon and talked about her visit home as they walked hand in hand through the park. It was a humid, hot summer day and they rested awhile in the ramada that overlooked the lake. The temptation was great with their seductive play and kisses that were held in check by the openness of the ramada. She assured him that everything was arranged for next Saturday and that he should plan to stay the night. Her aunt had visited her yesterday. There was an extra room and she said that it would be no imposition. He agreed and said that he would leave early in the morning, which would give her a day with her daughter, Carol, and her aunt.

A letter arrived that day from Bill Read in Phoenix, Arizona. The hot, dry desert climate agreed with him; his hay fever hadn't bothered him. It hadn't rained in Phoenix for a month. The days, he said, were clear and sunny with the temperature over 100. Sometimes it was over 110, but it was a dry heat and when it did rain, some of the people stood out in the rain like children watching the first snow of the season. Winter was the ideal time of the year and he invited Darrell to join the snowbirds and come to Arizona. He hadn't heard the term and thought snowbirds were like the wild geese from the north. Bill had a room at a boarding house on Third Avenue for thirty dollars a month, which included two meals a day except Saturday and Sunday. It was located within walking distance of downtown where he was a sales clerk in the men's department at Sears.

Darrell continued his walks in the afternoon and evening hours for a total of three hours of outdoor exercise a day. He met Patricia Brentwood on alternate afternoons and evenings as she was in class eight and permitted to be out walking an hour a day. It was the good old summertime and the walks were enjoyable. She was excited as she awaited a weekend visit home, the first in two years. She hadn't visited home sooner because she didn't want to expose Carol to any possible danger of being infected. Carol was five years of age and in two weeks she would be enrolled in kindergarten.

It was fun selecting records with Patricia that Saturday afternoon. The "Music Box" was busy and they didn't take time to play any of the records. Because of the numerous requests from the patients, both women and men, it was a process of elimination. Requests for some old favorites and songs that they could harmonize with predominated and included:

Harvest Moon,
Ah, Sweet Mystery Of Life,
The Way You Look Tonight,
I Don't Want To Walk Without You,
Ace In The Hole,
Ol' Man River,
Tales From The Vienna Woods,
In The Evening By The Moonlight,
Somebody Stole My Gal,

Five Foot Two,
Yes Sir, That's My Baby, and
Bye Bye Blues

Her aunt, "Wandering Wanda", Patricia called her, helped search for the records. She was tall with a very nice attractive personality and seven years older than Patricia who was thirty. She was working at a small factory on an electric motor assembly line and had sometimes traveled with her husband who was in the Marines until he was sent to the South Pacific.

They spent a delightful evening at her house. Martini cocktails were served before a light chicken dinner that was followed by a light mellow wine as they listened to some of the records. They were in a light mellow mood. After Carol was tucked in bed, he danced with Patricia until it was past time for them to retire. Wanda continued to pour the wine and insisted, over all his objections, that they would take him back to the hospital early in the morning.

He laughed and said that he only had "tee martunies" as he accepted another glass of wine and said that he wasn't accustomed to being treated so nice. He had called and scheduled a cab for early in the morning, which he then cancelled.

Patricia left to check on Carol and he danced with Wanda to the tune, The Way You Look Tonight as he gracefully thanked his hostess for a wonderful evening. When Patricia returned, they each had a nightcap before bidding each other goodnight.

Shortly after he had gone to bed the door opened ever so quietly and closed again. Patricia entered. "Are you asleep?"

"I'm not sleepy," he said as their hands met in the dark to a warm exciting touch. He led her into the bed beside him where his arms enfolded her and her nightgown slipped away.

The loving was wonderful and exciting with the gentle flowing momentum that had welled-up within to a strong responsive rhythm holding him firmly in a sensual, quivering, expansion of pleasurable satisfaction. They lay in each other's arms enjoying the pleasure of complete fulfillment.

"I've waited a long time for that," she whispered. "I didn't know I was capable after such a long time. I can sleep now," she said, slipping out of bed.

Wanda, who reminded him of his intention to return early, awakened him early in the morning. She said that Patricia was sleeping soundly. He told her not to wake her and that he would meet her on Monday for a walk in the park. It was a short, ten-minute drive and when they entered the circular drive by the men's building, a blue-pink dawn was breaking. As directed, she followed the drive to the nurses' building and made a wide turn back to the men's building. There was no one around when he got out near the rear entrance and with the box of records under his arm, he hurried in.

Darrell continued to take long walks to the golf course and the park, and on alternate afternoons and evenings he met Patricia Brentwood. His temperature had dropped to normal and he felt much better, and his concern for his empyema vanished when they were together. Their understanding for each other and their shared experiences made life wonderful with many adventurous thoughts of plans for future meetings. There was the realization that their love was for today with none of life's serious moments to mar their happiness. It was a life filled with youthful carefree dreams; a hopeful time when health was attainable once again.

Every two weeks his side was aspirated of the purulent fluid that was slowly diminishing, and then his pleural cavity was irrigated and cleansed with the Azocloramid solution. With the added exercise, his lung was expanding. Autumn arrived and he was scheduled for a series of tests and another X-ray. To date, all his cultures and tests were negative. He received his phrenic the last week of September. It was a relatively simple surgery and he was able to remain at the men's building. However, for two days his neck was stiff—so stiff that he could hardly turn his head. He met Patricia Brentwood for short walks around the hospital grounds. She thought he was funny the way he held his head erect and looked straight ahead. Even though the diaphragm on the right side of his chest was inactivated, there was no noticeable shortness of breath since his pleural wall had gradually thickened over the past year to protect his right lung. The small bandage and the stitches were removed four days later, leaving a narrow pink scar about an inch and a half long at the base of the neck, just above the right collar bone. That same day an X-ray was taken and blood was drawn from the vein of his arm for numerous blood tests, one of which was a sedimentation test.

He wrote a letter home and another to Bill Read about his progress and of his phrenic, and that he hoped to be released within a month.

Once again he began to take long walks with Patricia Brentwood along the lake and deep into the wooded area where they were alone and their friendship was enjoyable and more thrilling with each caress. She planned a visit home and he talked of his release and an uncertain future. The colorful autumn leaves were beginning to fall and the days were shorter. They knew that after many happy moments together along the trail, their walks would come to an end.

He anxiously awaited the results of his blood tests and his X-ray. A letter arrived from his sister, Mary. His mother was going to Good Samaritan Hospital for another X-ray. Mary planned to do some shopping in town on the seventeenth and would visit him.

Several days later he was fluoroscoped and 25 cc's of purulent fluid were drawn from the small pocket in his pleural cavity, and again, the pleural cavity was irrigated with the Azocloramid solution. He didn't like the looks of the fluid.

"Your fluid has decreased," said Doctor Sheridan. "In all

probability your fluid will disappear since your lung is about out. Your last X-ray was the same as your previous X-ray, which is good. How long have you been in class twelve?"

"Two and a half months."

"Have you taken your exercise?"

"Yes, two to three hours walking, almost every day."

"Your sedimentation test results were good and your sputum checks and cultures have been negative since a year ago last May."

"Will I be able to go home soon?"

"I believe you are able to keep regular hours and know enough to take care of yourself," said Doctor Sheridan. "You may go home next week if you like."

A happy, wonderful feeling overwhelmed him. He had waited a long time, almost two years, to hear those words, and now he could hardly believe it. His light blue eyes filled with tears.

"You have a good phrenic," continued Doctor Sheridan. "It will keep your lung partially at rest for ten to eleven months. Then you may need another phrenic. Furthermore, it is important for you to keep all the reserve breathing capacity that you have to maintain your health. Avoid places where the air is contaminated or polluted as much as possible, especially smoke filled rooms. A clean environment is essential for good health."

"Do you mean that I shouldn't smoke?"

"Yes, it is my opinion based on my experience, that smoking could damage your lungs. I wouldn't recommend it. Smoking certainly won't do your lungs any good. We don't have complete support of the community or all health agencies. It's a matter of common sense. I don't think that I can give you a set of rules to follow. Above all, don't worry. You have done well. Continue as you have been doing, and get proper rest and exercise."

"My sister will be visiting me on the seventeenth. I'll be going home then. It will be a surprise. And my thanks to you for all that you have done for me."

"How is your mother?"

"Her last X-ray was all right and she is having another one taken at Good Samaritan Hospital in Dayton, where Norma is in nurses' training."

The following week a special broadcast was arranged by the fellows at the new building—a secret, spur of the moment going home party. The lobby of the new building was filled with the women and men patients who were up in class. It looked as if all had turned out, even Miss Barnes, Miss Klingland and Mrs. Kenny stopped by. Patricia Brentwood did the announcing and Maw and Pap led them in the singing. Among the songs they sang were:

Roll Out The Barrel,
Sunny Side Of The Street,
Ace In The Hole,
Stay As Sweet As You Are,
Shine On Harvest Moon,
Three O'clock In The Morning,
Serenade In Blue,
You Are My Sunshine, and
Don't Get Around Much Anymore.

After the broadcast some of the fellows exercised the old player piano and the singing continued. There were stacks of rolls that had not been played in some time. Nine o'clock drew near. There was hand shaking and best wishes all around. He escorted Patricia to the elevator of the old building. There were tears of happiness in their eyes as they kissed good-bye, for the time that had been so long in coming was drawing near. They knew it had to be. It was the day they lived for, talked and dreamed about in their walks through the park, going home. She had planned a visit home the last weekend in October preceding his release. He accepted her invitation and planned to meet her there.

Chapter XXIV

HOME AND A CHANGING ATTITUDE

October 17, 1943, more than a year and eight months since he entered, Darrell bid farewell to his friends at the new building and life along "Commodilly Row" with its confining walls. What a grand and glorious feeling he had and he realized that the real test was about to begin as Doctor Sheridan had admonished. Mary was excited. She drove his '38 Chevy as if they didn't have time to get home. The back roads were familiar and there was little traffic. As much as he wanted to drive, he knew that he shouldn't overdo and that he couldn't do much of the farm work for some time—about five years based on the friendly advice of Doctor Sheridan. Mary was chatting away about the happenings at home. The home that his mother loved so much and had sacrificed for was sold by her mother to the Canning Company. Her father had built it and cleared the land. They had worked long and hard to save the farm during the depression years when his uncle had deserted it. Her mother lived with them for five years then left to be near her sons and daughters in Dayton. For Grandmother, there was too much noise and commotion, which at times did cause some conflict.

It was supper-time when they arrived home to a very unexpected but happy welcome. Except for Charles, who was in the army and Norma, who was in nurses' training, everyone was home. An extra place was added to the large dining room table making fifteen in all. Supper consisted of vegetables and fruit from the garden. Joe was talking with his father about the changes in the neighborhood. There had been several recent farm auctions. Many of the older families just packed up and sold the farm or rented out the fields and went to work in the nearby factories. He had rented and farmed 160 acres adjacent to the home place several years ago.

Joe remembered when he had gone threshing with the team of mules to help his dad during the summers of 1936 through 1939. It was dusty, hot and hard work but lots of fun to see who could haul the highest load. Sometimes there was an upset. The noon meals that were served were delicious and when the crop was extra good, there might be a keg of beer at the end of the long day's work. It had been a close, friendly neighborhood where each had to pull his share of the load at threshing time.

"The crops were good this year, but the pay wasn't that great," said Mr. Darrell. "We hired a combine to harvest the grain; that eliminates much of the work that was required by the old threshing machine."

"The Palmers are selling out and going to work in town at the furniture factory," said his mother.

"Yes, Tom Palmer is in his late fifties and he suddenly realized that after all the years on the farm, he had accumulated very little for his retirement. The farmers aren't covered by the Social Security program," said Mr. Darrell. "Let's finish our coffee in the parlor," he added as the girls were clearing the table. Both Mary and Ruth wanted to get the dishes washed and put away so that they could be ready when their dates arrived.

Their conversation continued in the parlor through the

evening hours. They told him that Mr. Crawley, an attorney who owned an adjacent sixty acre farm and a friend of his grandmother and family, had informed them in compliance with her instructions that the home place had been sold to the Canning Company. They had to comply. There was nothing that could be done. She was of sound mind, but influenced by Mrs. Darrell's brothers who had deserted the farm. After all they had done to save the home place, his grandmother sold out without talking to his parents. Joe thought of the summer vacations that he had spent with his grandmother and uncle working on the farm as a little boy. How could she do this to them at a time like this? They had ninety days to move, unless Mr. Darrell would work for the Canning Company. "I would only be paid the minimum wage which is forty cents an hour," his dad said, shaking his head. "I can't support the family on that. And if I use the tractor, I will get thirty cents an hour more which doesn't give me enough for gas." There was a pause. One of the little girls was crying in the kitchen. Several times they had looked in, as if to check on Mother. The little children were not allowed to play in the parlor. Most of the others were busy with their school books, and Mary and Ruth had left with their boyfriends.

"It's getting past their bedtime," said mother, rising to leave.

"And Joe, you don't want to overdo it on your first day."

"We'll continue our discussion tomorrow or at a later date.

We've got some planning to do," said his dad as they exchanged goodnights.

The sale of the home place had a tremendous impact on the family and the effects of things to come ran through his mind. He wondered what was to happen to the old farm equipment that occupied the west end of the barn including the old one-horse carriages. Also there was the spring buggy, the sleigh, an old Fordson tractor and there was a 1911 or 1912 four door Hudson with a high canvas top, as well as other antiques. Finally, he was overcome with sleep.

The morning air was clear and crisp as he helped his dad shuck some of the standing corn in the far field that he hoped to finish before the heavy snow came. His dad worked fast, shucking nearly two ears of corn to one for Joe whose hands were soft and tender from inactivity. Joe thought he might need gloves, but he managed. There was little talking, just a word now and then to the team of bay horses who seemed to know when it was time to pull ahead as they continued to flip the ears of corn into the wagon. When they came to the end of the rows where the field bordered a deep drainage ditch, his dad said they planned to move to a smaller farm where he could work in town and still do some farming. He liked farming and the open air better than factory work and he couldn't afford to work for the Canning Company. When Joe asked about all the old farm equipment, he was told that Mr. Crawley had informed them that there was to be an auction within ninety days or sooner and that he could include some of his items if he desired, but that there had to be an accounting of all items that belonged to grandmother.

He welcomed the afternoon rest hour and after three days of shucking corn, he was almost able to keep up. Within a week the corn harvest was complete.

Several days later he drove to Dayton for an interview with Mr. Cregor, the personnel manager at GM. After some discussion, he remembered the previous interview. Another X-ray was taken, and then there was a lengthy conference between the medical staff and personnel while Darrell waited patiently. He was alone in Mr. Cregor's office. A doctor entered carrying an X-ray and was followed by Mr. Cregor. Joe recognized the doctor from his previous physical.

"It is evident that you've had a considerable infection," said the doctor, pointing to the X-ray. "When were you released?"

"Last week," came Joe's cool response.

"You're fortunate in making the recovery as you have. I hope you understand that the company must consider all possibilities. We must consider the welfare of the other employees and students, and your chance of successful completion. We believe the training schedule, in conjunction with all the required work and outside study effort, would be too rigorous and not advisable for you to undertake."

"Even if you could not qualify for this program, time and youth are in your favor," said Mr. Cregor, eyeing him over the top of his spectacles and rubbing a hand through his snow-white hair as he continued. "It may help you to know that the company is supportive of better health services including preventive measures. The companies can't do it alone. We need more support from the government. Even the unions are against us sometimes."

There was a pause as they exchanged glances of intense compassion. "I can understand the company's position," said Darrell. "For more than a year I worked next to a fellow employee who previously had TB and when he broke down a second time, I wasn't concerned. Little did I realize how serious it was. I wasn't working with him at that time and I wasn't warned. I was working at Patterson Field then. If all companies required rigid physicals and exercised precaution including appropriate warnings, I would have been spared this disappointment."

He was appreciative of their help and consideration. There was no offer of employment and he had no desire to seek any other work at the moment. What would he do now when he could only work four hours a day. He had mixed emotions. He felt the agony of defeat and yet a sense of victory in that he had partially regained his health, however limited and guarded with a phrenic on his right lung. It was a changed life.

Enroute home, he drove slowly along Salem Avenue listening

to the car radio with thoughts of the future. He had about sixty dollars in poker winnings remaining. What could he do? It was then that he decided he had to go to Arizona and he would have to sell the car. He was saddened by the thought of selling his car. When he passed the street where Pat lived, his "Street of Dreams" he had called it, a hit tune on the radio with Peggy Lee singing seemed so appropriate:

"Somebody else is taking my place.
Somebody else now shares your embrace.
While I am trying to keep from crying,
you go around with a smile on your face."

Should he see Pat before he left? He wondered. He needed someone to talk to. He didn't feel at ease at home since he couldn't help with the work as he once had. He turned off Salem Avenue and stopped at Good Samaritan Hospital to visit Norma, his sister, who was in her second year of nurses' training. He told her about the interview and his decision to go to Arizona.

"I think it will be good for you," she said encouragingly. "I've heard that Joan, Bill Read's sister, has entered nurses training at St. Joseph's in Phoenix."

"I believe the drier climate will help me. How was Mother and Dad's last physical?"

"Both good. There wasn't any evidence that Mother ever had any TB infection. You need not be concerned or feel sorry."

"I believe the County Health Service forced Mother to spend three months at the sanatorium to be on the safe side. I couldn't understand why, but I feel much better about it now."

"We'll never know the reasons why; maybe it was a blessing in disguise."

Before he left the hospital he telephoned Pat. There was no answer and when he called the store where she worked, he was informed that she was on vacation. As he continued on his way home, he stopped at several car dealers to get some idea of the resale value. Cars were in demand. The highest offer received was $375.00, which was more than he had paid three years ago.

He didn't want to sell the car, but he could see no alternative. Automobile production facilities had been converted entirely to the war effort for the manufacture of tanks, airplanes, ships, guns and ammunition. Tires and gasoline were rationed. Women made up a large percentage of the work force. The whole world was in turmoil. The interview and the time spent in the sanatorium had left him with a sense of vulnerability. He had enjoyed competitive sports and now he realized that he could not participate physically.

That evening when he told his parents about the interview and his decision to go to Arizona, they expressed surprise and disappointment. Mr. Darrell's uncle, George, had gone west and wasn't heard from, and his father, John, was a millwright who had traveled the Ohio and Mississippi valley areas setting up machinery, including the alignment of pulleys and belts. John had wanted to go to Texas, but his wife didn't want to leave her sister and family relatives who had settled near Celina.

"Arizona...that's a long way from home. You'll have to go slowly and you must continue to take the afternoon rest hours," warned his mother.

"How will you go?" asked his dad.

"I plan to sell the car. I'll need the money. Then I'll hitchhike." After a pause Joe continued. "Maybe I'll take the train as far as St. Louis."

"That would be wise. You may run into some cold weather with rain and snow."

"Charles helped us to finish making the car payments," said his mother.

"I'll reimburse you when I sell the car. Charles got a lot of use out of it." Joe didn't want to sell his car. It had meant so much to him—the things he had done and the places he had gone. There was a shortage of cars and it would be worth more in Arizona, but he needed the money to get there.

His dad and mother exchanged glances and finally his dad said, "We can't afford another car. Your car does need new tires. Be careful when you drive." The tires were in good condition when he had examined them at Christmastime. Charles and his sisters really had put on the mileage.

That night he slept soundly. His mind was at ease; the decision was made. In the morning he wrote a letter to Bill Read telling him of his decision and that he would see him in about two weeks if he was lucky. He planned to hitchhike most of the way on Route 66 to Flagstaff and then on Route 89 through Sedona, Prescott and Wickenburg, and on to Phoenix. He asked him to arrange for a room where he was staying, if possible. The letter was sent airmail.

Later in the morning he took a walk through the woods where his dad was cutting wood. There were several large logs and he volunteered to help with the two-man cross-cut saw. Then they split the blocks of wood with the ax and wedges. His dad told him that he had heard from his sister, Minnie, who lived in Akron. She said that Goodyear was going to open a plant in St. Mary's, part of the war production effort, and manufacture rubber cleats or pads for tank tracks. In the twenties, when the family had moved to Dayton, he had worked for Dayton Rubber. There were several more days of wood cutting and working in the barn cleaning and oiling the farm implements.

On a Sunday evening, the last weekend in October, he kept his date with Patricia Brentwood. Sharing this evening together was wonderful as they talked about the change of events, his itinerary, and life in the far southwest. There was an air of excitement about him and in his arms she was excited, loving and lovable, knowing that this would be their last night together. On this night of lovemaking they were held in close embrace, filled with the enjoyment of loving and the desire of fulfillment that was theirs. It was enchanced by many long, lonely nights, long walks in the park, a shared similar experience, and an unknown future. She had four more months before her release from the sanatorium. They had learned the hard way the importance of a healthful diet, proper exercise and the importance of clean, clear air. Although prescription drugs might one day help to control this contagious plague, a healthy environment was most important. The night was still young when they exchanged goodnight kisses and good-byes, for tomorrow would be a busy day. The warm Indian summer weather was beginning to change.

For several days he visited the local car dealers and then the dealers in nearby towns. There wasn't much activity. Cars were scarce, but the dealers didn't want to pay much. During the week the weather turned colder with rain that changed to ice, then sleet and snow. The roads were hazardous and he spent a few days preparing for his trip west. He had an offer from a local dealer that he was considering. One afternoon, after rest hour, he hitched "Bud," one of the bay horses, to the sleigh and took a sleigh ride through the woods to pick up some of the wood that had been cut. The bay horse was fast and seemed to enjoy the snow. It continued to snow throughout part of the night. The next morning when the chores had been finished and the children were off to school, Mother and Dad joined him in another sleigh ride and they gathered more wood. It was a spur of the moment opportunity to be with his parents in a carefree, happy atmosphere. Mary, who was working the second shift at the local furniture factory, took care of the three pre-school girls. They were laughing and enjoying the sleigh ride as they talked about his journey to the far southwest. His dad said that it reminded him of his father's family who had come to this country in 1866 from Bavaria and settled in Cincinnati when his father, John, was ten years of age. His mother's family came from the northern part of Germany. She laughed as she talked about the differences in the languages—high German and low German. When Joe was a little boy his mother would sometimes speak in German if she didn't want him to know what they were talking about. Even his dad didn't always understand every word and sometimes he would respond in English. His mother said that they too would be moving in about two months. Mary Catherine (his mother used both names) had heard at one of the dances that there was a small, forty acre farm for sale near St. Marys. His dad added that it was just what they wanted and it wasn't far from the Goodyear plant. Mary and Ruth would help with the down payment.

Joe was surprised by the rapid change of events. "After all the years of hard work and sacrifice, you really deserve it. If you had told me before we started, I would have put the sleigh bells on Bud. When I sell the car, I'll contribute my share."

By midmorning the sun was breaking through the clouds and the weather turned warmer. The following morning he visited several of the local car dealers. It was only after some negotiation that he received a favorable offer including a ride home. What a sad, heart-breaking feeling he had as he watched his car disappear down the old graveled road. After he paid his parents two hundred and twenty-five dollars, the amount of the payments that had been made, he had one hundred and seventy-five dollars and eighty cents for his long journey west. Mother and Dad smiled proudly as they thanked him.

That afternoon he slept soundly for two hours, because sleep tonight on the train to St. Louis would be intermittent. From there he would take a bus out of town to Route 66 and hitchhike. Hopefully, the weather would be favorable as he was heading southwest. When he awoke, he finished packing his spare clothes in the small battered suitcase. The thoughts of leaving home left him with mixed emotions and sadness in his heart, and yet he felt it would be best for him.

Heartfelt wishes of good health and success were exchanged with his mother and dad. His dad presented him with a small, plastic-sealed "Sacred Heart" on a red background that was inscribed, "Peace!" and a Rosary saying, "These are for you. Use them faithfully. I will take you to the train depot."

It was a gray November day when he left home with high hopes for a new life in Arizona.

Chapter XXV

AN OVERNIGHT TRAIN TO ST. LOUIS

Following several blasts of the whistle, the train left Celina as Joe waved good-bye to his father. When the countryside became hidden in the dark of night, Darrell slept as best he could using a pillow from the luggage compartment above his coach seat. He was frequently jarred awake as stops were made at all towns enroute to St. Louis. A light tap on the shoulder awakened him and the conductor announced, "Last stop. St. Louis station." It was about six o' clock in the morning when he entered the large train depot and after inquiring about the local bus transportation, he ate a hearty breakfast at the restaurant. This was as far from home as he had ever traveled. What will the weather be like...and will I be lucky? he wondered as he boarded the local bus that eventually followed city Route 66 to the western edge of town.

The driver announced, "End of the line."

On the corner across the road from the bus stop was a large gas station and restaurant. Several trucks were parked there and he thought that perhaps he could get a ride west. No such luck. It was a cold, windy, overcast morning, but he was comfortable in his old raglan-sleeved overcoat as he stood by the side of the old battered suitcase along Route 66 heading west. Within a few minutes, a middle-aged fellow in an old pickup stopped and when Joe said that he was going to Arizona, he roared with laughter.

"I'm going to Rolla."

He didn't know exactly where Rolla was. "Where is Rolla?"

"That's only 100 miles down the road. I'll show you. This is the 'Show Me State'."

Joe smiled as he picked up his battered suitcase and jumped into the vacant seat of a 1936 Chevy pickup. Brief introductions were exchanged. Route 66 soon headed in a southwesterly direction through numerous small towns with cafes, stores, and gas stations. Some had tourist courts and garages that would be useful in an emergency. Harry who drove in an attentive, but carefree manner, through the small towns and rich farm country, mentioned points of interest. They passed the road to Meramec Cavern and north of Sullivan, Meramec State Park, consisting of hundreds of acres of beautiful natural forest with trails and cabins. As they approached Rolla, the overcast sky gave way to a bright, welcomed sun. According to Harry, the weather forecast was favorable with no rain. When he stopped for gas he told Joe that this was as far as he was going on Route 66 and he wished him luck on his trip to Arizona.

At Rolla he got a ride with Tom, a salesman in a 1940 Buick, who was going to Joplin. Leaving Rolla the highway became hilly, for they were traveling through the Ozarks. After about thirty miles, Tom pointed out Fort Leonard Wood, a large training center located to the right, and said that in his travels he had seen many a small town grow as a result of the training center and war effort. They were passing through Waynesville and he said it had become quiet a recreational town for the soldiers. The drive through Mark Twain National Forest was impressive with beautiful trees and some picnic tables alongside the highway.

From Lebanon to Springfield, Tom talked about the rolling hills, the beautiful streams and lake resorts. At times he slowed down as if he were going to stop, and once they were almost rear-ended by a large semi-truck. Joe was concerned. Tom was in his sixties and he did appear tired. Joe asked if he wanted to rest while he drove. Tom said that he was alright, but as they approached Springfield, he suggested that Joe drive as the rest sounded good and it would give him a chance to prepare for his sales meeting in Joplin. As directed, Joe took Bypass 66 and when checking the gauges he noted that they were low on gas.

"No problem," said Tom. "Pull off at the next exit."

It was touch and go as they coasted along. The gas gauge showed empty when they reach a gas station and filled up. From Springfield, Route 66 was less hilly with less winding curves and Joe made better time. Gas stations and garages were only a few miles apart. Just west of the Joplin business district, Tom took control and Joe was on his own again. It was about 12:30 P.M. He had made good time—about 300 miles since he left St. Louis. He ate a good lunch at a nearby restaurant and then with his coat and luggage in hand, he walked along the road to a large park where he stood momentarily to admire the view. After a while he turned to face the west-bound traffic. There really weren't many cars. After a short while a 1940 Ford convertible came into view and he raised his right thumb high. To his surprise it stopped in front of him and as he walked up to the passenger side, a young lady leaned over and asked, "How far are you going?"

"Phoenix, Arizona," he replied with a big smile. "How far are you going?" he asked picking up his coat and suitcase.

"Los Angeles, California. You may put your luggage behind the front seat," she said as she unlocked the door. "I'm Betty Blake from Rochester, New York."

"Glad to meet you. I'm Joe Darrell from Celina, Ohio."

Betty was twenty-six with light brown hair and attractive.

She said that she was going to Los Angeles to be with her friend who was in a hospital, and that he was in the Air Force and had been wounded fighting in the Pacific.

"Were you in the service?" asked Betty.

He told her that he had spent eighteen months in a sanatorium and that he had been released about a month ago. Their conversation was interrupted at times with comments on the scenery. They passed some huge mounds of tailings from lead and zinc mines and crossed the Missouri-Kansas state line and the Eagle-Picher Co. It was a short drive through this southeast section of Kansas and less than twenty miles through Galena, Riverton and Baxter Springs. When they reached the Kansas-Oklahoma state line, she asked if he had a driver's license and said that she had stayed in Terre Haute, Indiana last night. When he told her that he did have a valid Ohio driver's license, she stopped on the shoulder of the road where they exchanged seats. Before he pulled onto the highway, he pulled out his billfold to show her his license.

"Oh, I believe you! You don't need to show me."

"There isn't much money in it," he said and as she looked at his driver's license more out of curiosity, he added, "about seven dollars."

"You're going to Arizona on seven dollars?"

"I guess I can tell you. I've got about $150 in my socks to tide me over until I find work. I had to sell my '38 Chevy to pay my debts. I really didn't want to, but I needed the money.

"In your socks," she laughed. "I got a hundred in my bra." And after he had pulled onto the highway, she said, "Don't drive more than sixty."

There was more evidence of mining activity, but soon the hills were lower and less frequent and they were heading into a strong southwesterly wind. At sixty miles per hour the noise of blowing wind was quite noticeable, even though the top of the convertible was up and the windows were closed. When they passed through the town of Claremore, Betty mentioned that it was the home of Will Rogers, and continued, "Before we were interrupted, I wanted to ask why you were in a sanatorium for eighteen months?"

"I had tuberculosis."

"How did you get that? And how old are you?"

"I'll be twenty-two next month. For a year I worked next to a fellow who had tuberculosis and never knew it, and didn't realize how serious it was. Eight months later, after I had worked at Patterson Field in Dayton Ohio, an X-ray was taken when I applied for an engineering training program at General Motors. The climate in Arizona should be better for me and as the saying goes I'll take it 'one day at a time' and enjoy a new life. I now realize that good health and environment means everything. A very good friend who was released from the sanatorium two years ago is working in Phoenix."

Near the outskirts of Tulsa, as he reached the crest of a hill, several children were playing in the middle of the highway. He blasted the horn, applied the brakes and they literally flew toward the shoulder of the road. No cars were approaching as he swerved around them. Betty slumped on his shoulder. In Tulsa they stopped for gas and Betty drove. There were many oil wells there and a railroad ran alongside Route 66 at times. The road passed though a rolling countryside and many oil derricks were visible. They by-passed Oklahoma City and when she stopped at a tourist court at El Reno, she said, "We'll spend the night here. You register."

He was momentarily taken by surprise. "What would you like? Adjoining rooms?"

"That would be fine."

He registered and they looked at the assigned rooms, which were neat and clean, each with a double bed, and there was one adjoining bathroom. He offered to pay his share, but she wouldn't accept. He did pay for dinner at a nearby restaurant and when they returned to their rooms, they both took a shower and retired early. As he lay in bed he didn't feel sleepy. Many thoughts of the day ran through his mind and when he heard some stirring in the adjoining room, he called out, "I'm not sleepy," and Betty leaped into bed beside him. They hugged and kissed and as her legs spread he rolled on top. After some attempts to enter, she guided him into a world of sensational loving, and with gasps of excitement, she folded her legs over his. In rhythmical muscular action they reached their climax in unison. After more hugging and kissing, she left to sleep alone in her room. Early in the morning she awakened him and another terrific lovemaking session followed.

Leaving El Reno, Route 66 passed through ranch country with many stone picnic tables along the roadway. Betty was driving and the first stop was Elk City for gas and a short drive around some of the red brick streets that had tall elm trees and beautiful homes. It reminded him of Celina, Ohio. The road headed southwest through Sayre and across a fork of the Red River. He thought of the song Red River Valley. At the western towns of Erick and Texola, the road turned directly west to the Texas-Oklahoma state line where she asked him to take over.

It was a pleasant sunny day and the road crossing the Panhandle was good. They passed rich oil fields and after the town of Shamrock rows of trees, which served as windbreakers. When they reached the Plains, there were very few trees and any visible ranches were a great distance apart. The noise of the blowing wind along the top of the convertible was annoying at times and still sounded in his ears whenever he slowed down or stopped, but he wasn't too concerned as the convertible was in good condition. At Amarillo they had lunch and filled up with gas.

He was able to hold a fairly steady speed and after seventy-five miles, they entered New Mexico at Glenrio. The road was rough and at Tucumcari the terrain changed. Steep cliffs appeared in the distance beyond the dry plateau countryside. The time zone changed from Central to Mountain Time and they set their watches back an hour. The road climbed at times through the rugged picturesque country that had served as a hide-away for some early cattle rustlers. At Santa Rosa he stopped for gas and Betty drove. He sat back and relaxed as they talked about the country and Route 66. He mentioned The Grapes of Wrath by John Steinbeck. It was a story of Okies going out to California as a result of the dust bowl and the depression of the 1930's. Other stories and songs were commented on...such as Drifting Along with a Tumbling Tumbleweed. Many had been seen blowing across the road. Mountains in the far distance came into view and there were stretches of steep climbs and then the road wound down through Tijeras Canyon to Central Avenue in Albuquerque. There were several trading posts that sold Indian jewelry, woven blankets, baskets and curios from nearby Indian reservations. She stopped at a tourist court in the center of town. It was late in the afternoon. She told him to register and they decided on one room. When they entered the room she immediately jumped onto the double bed and with laughter, she said that it was a good firm mattress. He joined in the laughter and as he approached, she said, "Let's shower and eat first."

After dinner they walked around town and visited an exhibit of Indian antiques near the Santa Fe railroad station. Along Central Avenue they passed Indians in native costumes. Although this was mid-November, it was a pleasant evening that was beginning to cool rapidly as the sun set in the west. A most pleasant, enjoyable night was spent together sharing a thrilling night of love. They each enjoyed a high climax together with lingering kisses. They slept soundly and were awakened by a wake-up call. She had a schedule to meet and there was a lot to see and do on the route to Flagstaff. From there he planned to go to

Phoenix and sometimes he thought it would be a good chance to go to Los Angeles. After breakfast they stopped for gas and when they crossed the Rio Grande River, the sun was beginning to rise in the east. Heading west there were many tourist courts and stores, and beyond the western suburbs the highway began to climb out of the Rio Grande valley up Nine Mile Hill. The morning sun reflected on the Sandia Mountain Peaks and a few scattered clouds over the city of Albuquerque. After several long hills and valleys, the road passed through high mesa country with flat-top mountains in the distance that had been used by the Indians to build their adobe homes and Pueblos. There were some small villages with trading posts, curios, stores and gas stations. Just west of Santa Maria, a large area of ancient lava flow was visible on both sides of the highway. She said that this was called the "Malpais" which means the badlands.

"How did you know that?" he asked.

"This is my second trip and I tried to read about the route. I've seen some of the Indian dances. At home I've danced until the early morning hours; I've danced the night away."

"Do you like to dance?"

"Oh yes! But I'm a little out of practice."

At Grants the landscape changed to ranch and farmland, and she called his attention to the green fields, acres and acres of carrots, and said that most of the work was done by the Indians. It was all hand labor and shipped east by railroad. There were little round houses for the workers, which she called, "Navajo Hogans."

"You do know a lot about this part of the country."

"I've spent some time in Albuquerque when my friend was stationed there at the air base. That was just a little more than a year ago, in 1942."

"Did you go to any of the Indian dances?"

"Yes, we enjoyed them."

He could detect an emotional change as she talked about her friend who had been wounded, and there were times when she was driving much faster now through small communities with trading posts. Soon they crossed the Continental Divide, which was more than 7,000 feet in elevation and there was a gradual decline past red sandstone cliffs and then into Gallup. It was a major railroad center and leading Indian trade center with arts and crafts from the surrounding reservation. At Gallup, they stopped for gas and changed drivers. She had complete trust in him, which was evident in their discussions and actions. The maroon convertible was performing well. He was tempted to stop at the El Rancho Motel, but he knew that her time was limited. After twenty-five miles they crossed the Arizona state line and a border inspection. In the trunk along with the luggage were two-gallon jugs and a smaller one in the back by his suitcase.

"What is in the jugs? What is your destination?" asked the inspector.

"California, and there's water in the jugs," Betty said.

"You're wise to carry extra water in the desert. Proceed."

It was a high, dry desert with a few villages. Some had a trading post, gas station and cafe. They had lunch at Navajo and then stopped at an observation pull-off where they had a good view of the Painted Desert—a colorful expanse of rocky soil in shades of yellow, rose, blue and purple, that extended into the horizon. On the left, a side road led to the Petrified Forest that consisted of thousands of acres where they enjoyed a walk among the colorful petrified logs. Occasionally he stopped to feel the logs and small pieces scattered about and she warned him that he could only touch. He agreed. He never had any such intentions although it was tempting. Following a short visit to the museum, they returned to Route 66 and continued west through Holbrook and Joseph City. At Winslow he pulled in for gas and Betty took over. A brief stop was made at Meteor Crater, a huge hole about three miles around and about six hundred feet deep. In the distance the snow-capped San Francisco Peaks were visible and she said, "That's near Flagstaff where you want to get off."

"Where will you be staying tonight?" He thought perhaps they could spend another night together after a visit to the Grand Canyon.

It was mid-afternoon and she said that she would be staying at Needles, California and would have stopped at Flagstaff, but this was her menstrual period and she was beginning to menstruate. A calm, thoughtful expression covered her face as she momentarily glanced at him.

"It has been a wonderful trip and the weather has been great. I really don't want to get off at Flagstaff."

"That would be your best route to Phoenix; a scenic, well-traveled route."

The road entered the Coconino National Forest with tall pines, and after passing Winona, a trading center, the road began a steady climb into Flagstaff where the elevation was about 7,000 feet. In town she stopped at a convenient hotel and as they began to exchange farewells, she asked for his full name and the address of his friend in Phoenix where he planned to stay. He wrote his name and address on her note pad and with heartfelt thanks he stepped out and waited. She waved and her blue eyes twinkled as she drove away.

In the hotel lobby he read some of the pamphlets. There was the Museum of Northern Arizona, the Lowell Observatory, the Sante Fe Railroad, and the bus service, which could take him to the Grand Canyon. He had seen a bus station less than a block away and as he walked to the station, he noticed a shortness of breath, the effects of the high altitude, his phrenic and one lung to go. Rather than spend the night there he decided to take a bus to Phoenix. It was after four o'clock when he left the city in the tall pines, the lumber mills and the lofty peaks in the clear blue sky, via alternate 89 leading into Oak Creek Canyon. From the window of the bus, a series of hairpin curves or switchbacks could be seen. At one time in the descent from the Mogollon Rim, he counted seven and the view was breathtaking. The eroded canyon walls were brilliant with shades of red, gray, green and white with the contrasting autumn leaves of the cottonwood, sycamore, oak and maple. Oak Creek Canyon was magnificent and a well constructed road twelve miles in length ran along a crystal clear mountain stream. Its walls were 2,500 feet and three miles wide at the lower end where the colorful, red rock cliffs and Sedona came into view. There were some orchards and a few ranch houses, a country store, trading post, tiny post office and a small motel in Sedona. The bus made a brief stop and he got off to stretch. In the hotel lounge there was a party. One cowboy with a guitar was singing Back In The Saddle Again. Several couples dressed in western clothes, boots, blue jeans and broad-rimmed hats were dancing. All were having a great time. Three couples left with the bus that continued on alternate 89 through the Verde Valley and Sycamore Canyon regions with brief stops at Cottonwood and Clarkdale. Here several miners boarded the bus for the mining town of Jerome. In the twilight, many houses could be seen high on the mountainside; many were on stilts. Jerome was an old copper mining town. The view from the windows of the bus down into the steep canyons at Jerome were scary at times. When the bus arrived at Prescott, it was almost dark. Prescott was the first capital of Arizona; a mile high city located in a bowl-shaped valley with the Bradshaw Mountains and tall pines on the south and west. There was a half-hour layover there and he had a light supper at a restaurant on "Whiskey Row", a famous street across from the large Yavapai County Courthouse. There on a cement plaza, a square dance was in progress. There were six squares all having a great time swinging to the caller's cues and the western songs. This was unusual for mid-November, but the weather was very mild.

Leaving Prescott, the mile high city with attractive, historical homes, Highway 89 headed southwest over a very winding road. The couple in the seat ahead of him were counting the curves and said there were more than ninety-three. The road straightened through Wilhoit, Kirkland, Peeple's Valley, large cattle ranch country, and on to Yarnell, about thirty-five miles distance. From the top of Yarnell Hill, Highway 89 was a long, winding, steep downgrade along the mountainside for about eight miles and then straight to Congress Junction. They went on to Wickenburg, a small western town, famous for its dude ranches. At the bus station, a rancher and an old prospector welcomed the passengers with a "Howdy" and a song...long long ago...the horses ask. The cows ask...All ask for you...long ago...long long ago... Several cowboys and cowgirls got off the bus amid the roaring laughter and high spirits. There was a western dance celebration going on at the dude ranches.

Route 89 from Wickenburg toward Phoenix followed along the Hassayampa River. There were only a few vacant seats on the bus. Darrell relaxed with thoughts of his arrival in Phoenix and the future. It was a great unknown, but youth was in his favor and Bill Read had encountered the same situation two years ago after having spent two and a half years in the sanatorium before his release. Bill would be a great help, he thought. Luck was with him and it had been a great trip west. His thoughts drifted as the road passed small communities where the ranch land and desert terrain became transformed via desert cultivation with cotton, alfalfa, vegetables and citrus groves that existed along the northern Salt River Valley, leading passed Glendale and to Phoenix.

The bus station, which was located on Jefferson Street, a half block east of Central Avenue, was crowded. It was eight-thirty in the evening. He walked to the Jefferson Hotel at Central and Jefferson where he called Bill Read. Bill had received his letter, but had not expected him for another week. As luck would have it, there was a bed available where Bill resided.

He had a grand, wonderful feeling as he awaited a taxi. It was a pleasant warm night and there was a slight breeze blowing. This was mid-November. He was indeed happy to be in Arizona.